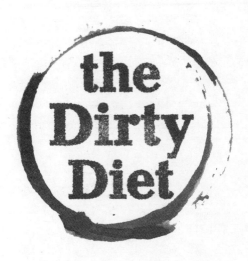

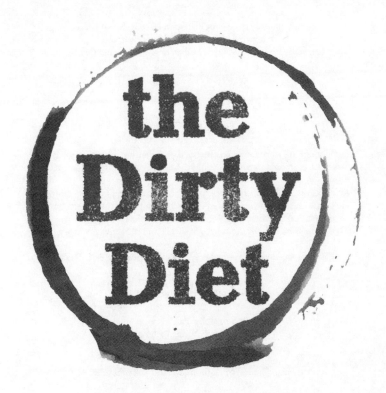

the Dirty Diet

Ditch the guilt, love your food

KATE HARRISON

SEVEN DIALS

First published in Great Britain in 2018 by Seven Dials
An imprint of Orion Publishing Group Ltd
Carmelite House, 50 Victoria Embankment, London, EC4Y 0DZ

An Hachette UK Company

1 3 5 7 9 10 8 6 4 2

Text © Kate Harrison 2018

A CIP catalogue record for this book is available from the British Library.

Paperback ISBN: 9781409171287
Ebook ISBN: 9781409171294

Photography: Faith Mason
Food stylist: Nicola Richman
Prop stylist: Rebecca Newport

Printed and bound CPI Group (UK) Ltd, Croydon, CR0 4YY

Every effort has been made to ensure the information in this book is accurate.
The information in this book may not be applicable in each individual case so
it is advised that professional medical advice is obtained for specific health
matters and before changing any medication or dosage. Neither the publisher
nor author accepts any legal responsibility for any personal injury or other
damage or loss arising from the use of the information in this book. In addition
if you are concerned about your diet or exercise regime and wish to change
them, you should consult a health practitioner first.

Every effort has been made to fulfil requirements with regard to reproducing
copyright material. The author and publisher will be glad to rectify any
omissions at the earliest opportunity.

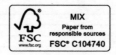

www.orionbooks.co.uk

Contents

Welcome to the Dirty Diet   7

Health advice and caution   21

Part 1: Dirty Diet Principles   23

The principles behind the Dirty Diet   25

Part 2: Your Dirty Diet Blueprint   79

3 steps to creating your Dirty Diet blueprint   81

    First stage: you today   83

    Second stage: you in the future   89

    Third stage: your action plan   98

Blueprint examples   106

My Dirty Diet blueprint   110

Part 3: The Dirty Diet Plans and Recipes   113

The plans and the recipes   115

We ♥ fruit and veg   118

The meal plans   124

A note on calorie-counting   146

Dirty Diet Recipes — 148

   Breakfasts and brunches — 149

   Soups and light meals — 173

   Main dishes — 199

   Main dishes + — 246

   Side dishes and sweet things — 254

Quick calorie counter and ideas for Dirty Diet-friendly foods — 270

Probiotic foods — 279

Choosing ready-made meals and prepared foods — 299

Eating out and takeaway guidance — 304

Part 4: Dirty for life — 313

Supplements — 318

Exercise and weight loss — 326

How to keep a two-day food diary — 329

You and your microbes – friends for life — 332

The future of microbiome, personalised weight loss
and longevity research — 338

Resources — 341

Index — 355

Acknowledgements — 360

Your questionnaire — 362

The Dirty Diet made simple — 366

Welcome to the Dirty Diet.

Ditch the guilt. Love your food. Lose weight for good.

Do you want to lose up to 15 lbs (7 kg) in 28 days, without giving up your favourite foods or feeling guilty? Would you love a fuss-free plan that doesn't tell you food is bad or 'naughty', but focuses on how enjoyable eating well can be? An approach that gives you the benefits of the latest research on longevity, brain health and gut science?

Then the Dirty Diet is for you.

Forget clean eating, neurotic obsessions and unscientific rules, which have become all too familiar to weary dieters. Instead, enjoy all the foods you love: cheese, full-fat yogurt, carbs including bread and grains, fresh produce, meat and fish (if you like them), plus coffee and wine. Real, tasty food. Nothing banned. And no more guilt . . . Because as I'm about to show you, eating well is all about variety, not restriction, and about focusing on what makes *you* feel and look your best.

In only four weeks, people who tried out the Dirty Diet lost up to 15lbs (7kg); dropped two dress sizes; saw great improvements in their mood and gut health; and found a plan they can enjoy for life. And don't just take my word for it – here's what our participants said:

I have lost 15 lbs (7 kg) after 28 days. The Dirty Diet is the best diet I've ever been on, which sounds like hyperbole but is honestly what I feel. I like the fact that it's not faddy. I like the expertise behind it. I love the fact that it doesn't preach. I've failed at all other diets I've tried before, including seeing a hospital dietitian. This is the first diet that made sense because there is so much emphasis on me as an individual. I don't have to fit into a one-size-fits-all way of living.

Bridget, 62, tutor and writer from Brighton, UK

Over the four weeks, I lost 14 lbs (6.3 kg), which I was really surprised and pleased by. I also noticed I slept better, had no acid reflux, and my psoriasis was much less itchy and annoying. I also have more energy. Best of all, it's been easy for me to adopt as a lifestyle, and has really stuck.

Rose, 46, lecturer from Hertfordshire, UK

I'm 10 lbs (4.5 kg) down in 28 days and I feel so much healthier; it's working better than any other diet I've ever tried. Not only has it allowed me to change my eating habits and expand the range of the foods I enjoy – I really feel better about myself.

Quinton, 27, IT technician from Durban, South Africa

I lost 12.5lbs (5.6kg) in four weeks and I'm over the moon – I can't believe how much better I feel in myself. I'm sleeping better, my IBS has settled down a lot, and I've rediscovered enjoyment of food rather than just eating for the sake of eating, as well as a few new favourite recipes! It makes a lovely change to eat yummy food and not feel guilty about enjoying it.

Jenni, 36, office administrator from Warwickshire, UK

I lost 12lbs (5.5kg) in 28 days: I am proud of my achievements and feel that I can, for the first time in over 20 years, reach my ideal weight this way. I felt so lost, knowing I need to lose weight to be around for my eight-year-old daughter, knowing my eating was killing me, but feeling so overwhelmed by all the different diets. Should I eat clean, should I eat Paleo, or low-carb? Then I tried the Dirty Diet and I feel liberated!

Sarah, 42, deputy principal, Perth, Australia

I am beyond excited. I'm down two dress sizes and have had compliments from my mother-in-law! After having tried so many diets – of which many worked but were not sustainable – this is the one for me. The diet (scratch that – lifestyle!) is easy and, more importantly, sustainable.

Patricia, 52, translator from Quebec, Canada

What *is* the Dirty Diet?

It's a simple, personalised plan that will help you lose weight, improve your health, and ditch any guilt you feel for eating food you love. It's both flexible and sustainable: this book contains all you need for the first four weeks – and the rest of your life. When you decide to eat dirty, you will:

- **Lose weight** and feel in the best shape, physically and mentally;
- **Ditch the guilt** and fall back in love with real food (including easy, quick options for busy lives);
- **Eat in tune with the latest nutritional research**, reaping benefits from game-changing work on fasting and the gut microbiome.

Is the Dirty Diet for me?

Yes, if:

- You want to lose weight in a sustainable, enjoyable way – and keep it off;
- You want to improve your diet without any faddy restrictions or half-baked theories;
- You want simple, delicious meals that benefit gut health and mood;
- You'd like to find practical ways to benefit from the latest nutritional research.

On top of all that, people who have already tried the Dirty Diet also reported improvements in digestion; better sleep; more energy; lower anxiety levels; improvements in acne, eczema and rosacea; fewer cravings and blood sugar fluctuations; and the pleasure of enjoying a more balanced, diverse and satisfying diet!

How does the Dirty Diet work?

The Dirty Diet works by offering easy, flexible meal plans and simple guidelines you can stick to for life. The approach includes Plenty Days and Fast Days:

Plenty Days: 4–5 days per week

On Plenty Days, you'll choose three delicious meals – including easy-to-prepare recipes and ready-made options – adding up to **1800 calories** per day (with some flexibility depending on how quickly you're aiming to lose weight).

ON THE MENU: You could be tucking in to bubble-and-squeak with egg at breakfast, a vegetable balti at lunchtime, and smoked salmon and gruyère tart or mushroom and leek risotto for dinner, washed down with a glass of red wine.

Fast Days: 2–3 days per week

On Fast Days, you'll enjoy lower-calorie meals, which are still nutritious and filling and include lots of veg, adding up to a daily total of **600–750 calories**. As well as producing weight loss, these lighter days help retune your appetite *and* benefit your health by encouraging cell renewal and recycling.

ON THE MENU: You could be eating a yogurt granola sundae with strawberries for breakfast, minestrone with pesto for lunch and Middle Eastern lamb meatballs or avocado Caesar salad for dinner.

You'll find vegetarian and meat/fish options for both Plenty Days and Fast Days. **Nothing is banned**, including alcohol and 'treats', but you'll eat an increased variety of foods, with more vegetables, fruit, grains, fibre and whole foods including cheese, full-fat live yogurt, nuts and seeds. **Snacking is strongly discouraged** – but with our super-filling dishes you won't need to eat between meals! And don't worry if time or money are short: your choices include ready-made, great value meals as well as home-made dishes.

How does this equal weight loss?
The **Fast Days** help you achieve the calorie gap or deficit you need to lose weight – while making you aware of how filling and tasty healthy food can be.

The **Plenty Days** are about balance, variety and flavour, with nutritious, tasty ingredients, plus a little of what you fancy . . . including foods that other diets ban. The flexibility is what makes this plan so sustainable. You will want to live this way for good!

Why 'dirty'?
Because eating should be fun, pleasurable and messy – not clean, sterile and obsessive. So many diets seem to want to punish us for having an appetite! Yet it makes no sense to ban the real, unprocessed foods we've loved for centuries, including fresh bread, salted butter, strong cheese, eggs, vegetables, plus tasty meat and fish if you're not a vegetarian.

Who doesn't want a picnic on the beach, with crispy salad and the catch of the day grilled on a bucket barbecue? Or a breakfast with food from the farm gate: freshly picked spinach, flash-fried field mushrooms, bread still warm from the oven, served with blue-veined cheese or full-fat yogurt? Or a family lunch of free-range roast chicken with all the trimmings, followed by crumble made with windfall apples and brambles from the Sunday morning walk?

Dirty is *not* a dirty word when it comes to ingredients. The food we're celebrating is:

- **Fresh and dirty** – that doesn't rule out all prepared foods, but it focuses on food that's at its peak.
- **Good and dirty** – packed with nutrients and the good bacteria that aid mental and physical health.
- **Quick and dirty** – unfussy dishes, easy to prepare.
- Above all, it's **delicious and dirty** – flavour comes first.

I believe no food is 'good' or 'evil'. Food isn't punishment or religion – it's nourishment. Excess can be bad for you, yes, but the less you obsess, the more likely you are to listen to your body and **eat a balanced diet**, while losing weight or maintaining a healthy shape.

And that's what the Dirty Diet is all about.

The dirty truth about clean eating

Crucially, this plan is the OPPOSITE of 'clean eating'. If you haven't heard the term, clean eating is an approach that recommends cutting out entire food groups – from wheat to dairy to coffee and even some vegetables. It's claimed these ingredients make us ill, and avoiding them will make us well again.

Of course, food allergies and intolerances *do* exist. But for most of us, an extreme exclusion diet isn't healthy or sustainable. Obsessing over supposed toxins or hidden dangers can lead to expensive food bills and nutritional deficiency – it may also encourage orthorexia nervosa, an unhealthy obsession with food that defies logic and evidence.

The other problem with excluding major food groups – as Paleo and low-carb approaches also advocate – is it's REALLY hard to stick to. I've seen it lead to obsessive behaviour, and terrible guilt or stress when someone 'falls off the wagon'. Anyone can stick to a highly restrictive diet for a few days, weeks, even months. But sooner or later, you are likely to give in to cravings.

Healthy eating is about balance, not bans

That doesn't mean everything about clean eating is wrong – there's often an emphasis on healthy fresh vegetables, for example. But it's not a diverse approach. I don't want to live a life without fresh bread and butter, a glass of red wine with a meal, blue cheese, a bowl of pasta, a hot curry and basmati rice, strong espresso coffee with a chocolate truffle, Italian ice cream on a hot day . . . the list is endless. Good food makes the good times even better.

If you have an allergy, or coeliac disease, you do need to take special care. But for most of us, eating diversely across the main food groups will make us feel great, and reduces our risk of bingeing on 'forbidden foods'.

Diversity also ensures you're getting a wide range of the macronutrients and micronutrients that are essential to physical *and* mental health, as we'll see later on in the book.

Who am I and why this plan?

I'm the author of the bestselling 5:2 Diet series – five books about intermittent fasting that have sold around the world. I invented the Dirty Diet after taking stock of what I've learned from writing those books. Since I first started writing I've talked to tens of thousands of people who want to transform their health and weight, and the Facebook group I set up in 2012 to share tips with a few friends now has 60,000 members. Every day, I interact with people who want to lose weight and feel better, and it's given me an insight into what works best and the information dieters need. Essentially, the Dirty Diet was designed to meet their needs – and yours – by including:

- **Advice about Plenty Days, as well as Fast Days.** Many people find the Fast Days simple enough, but want much more guidance on eating the rest of the time, and staying well long term.
- **The know-how to nurture your microbes as well as yourself.** As people in my group posted their fantastic before and after photos, and celebrated success, I struggled to understand why some people were finding it so much easier to lose and maintain weight than others. In 2014, I started reading research on the gut microbiome – our own personal

colony of trillions of bacteria – and I realised they may hold the key to health in so many areas, including our weight. Encouraging the good bacteria to thrive – through delicious foods and positive habits – is an essential part of this plan.

- **Ways to personalise the plan to fit your needs, goals and tastes.** One size never fits all. Diets that have strict rules fail most of the time. So in the Dirty Diet, you create a personalised version that suits your needs, tastes and goals. Whether you want to lose 7 lbs before an event, or kick off a major weight loss goal that will transform your health, you set the pace, choose the meals, and select mental strategies to keep you on track.

As well as my Facebook members and readers, the Dirty Diet has also been inspired by my own journey – nearly six years after starting to cut back only two days a week, I'm 2 stone lighter and I've maintained that healthy weight for the first time in my adult life: and despite a strong family history of type 2 diabetes, my HbA1c levels (a measure of blood sugar levels over time) are so good my GP had to check twice. Keeping the weight off has been about embracing my favourite foods, trying new ingredients (you'll read about my sometimes explosive exploits later) and studying research on what works.

Introducing Helen

I've worked with registered dietitian and sports nutrition consultant **Helen Phadnis** to ensure the Dirty Diet is right up-to-date with the latest science – but in a simple, easily digestible form. Helen and I have compared notes over strong coffee – which she loves as much as I do – to create a plan that not only offers weight loss, but also brings huge health benefits. She'll be adding her expertise throughout the book.

Helen's background working in the NHS and with private clients has proved invaluable. As she says:

In hospitals, I saw the healing power of optimal nutrition on a daily basis – from counselling kidney failure patients on how to slow the progression of their disease through diet, to calculating the exact artificial nutrition preparation for those patients with complete gut failure.

After further training, I started up private practice within sports nutrition. My private practice has expanded to include diet counselling for irritable bowel syndrome and weight management, as well as sports performance. The key to optimising health or weight and sporting goals is to focus on habits and foods to introduce into your diet, not on those that should be cut out.

The Dirty Diet doesn't just help those trying to lose weight: it will help those wanting to boost their mood, immunity, sporting performance; it's for people who would like to sleep better, reduce bloating, not feel hungry all the time. It's designed to encourage **health gains** *in addition to weight loss, and that is what I love about it.*

How the book works

Part 1 – Dirty Diet Principles: the science and psychology behind the Dirty Diet

D is for **Diverse diet** – eating a wide range of ingredients, especially fresh vegetables, dairy, wholegrains, nuts and high-quality proteins. This diversity means you're getting a wider spectrum of nutrients and lots of fibre – while 'smart harvesting' foods allow you to eat more and still lose weight.

I is for **Intermittent fasting** – limiting your calorie intake on certain days helps you lose weight and become aware of healthy choices. Fasting helps the body to do essential maintenance, and makes us aware of appetite signals – including when we're full!

R is for **Restoring gut health** – promoting good digestion, immunity and mood by eating the right live foods (probiotics) and fibre (prebiotics). There are astonishing connections between gut and general health, brain function and weight.

T is for **Training yourself in healthy habits** to encourage a long and active life. I know how hard it can be to change poor habits, even if you *really* want to. We give you practical tools to address cravings, trigger foods and motivations.

Y is for **You** – customising the diet to suit your energy needs, likes and dislikes, and weight loss or health goals.

Part 2 – Your Dirty Diet Blueprint: your goals, your choices, your success

This stage is all about the Y in Dirty – You! Answer simple questions to fit this plan to your exact requirements.

- **Your needs**: your calorie needs on a weekly and daily basis
- **Your goals**: for weight loss, health, mental outlook
- **Your likes and dislikes:** food that suits you
- **Your motivation:** what you want, why you want it, and how to achieve it

This section allows you to create your own Dirty Diet Blueprint to reach your health and weight goals.

Part 3 – The Dirty Diet Plan and Recipes: Steady and Speedy meal plans, plus recipes

This section contains everything you need to get results on the Dirty Diet Steady and Speedy eating plans which have given our dieters losses of up to 15 lbs (7 kg) in 28 days – both plans stick to the same principles, but the number of Fast Days and calorie limits are different depending on your needs. In keeping with Part 2, you can personalise all the plans to create your own perfect Dirty Diet.

Plus, try out 50+ delicious tried and tested recipes. There's also advice on choosing prepared meals and eating out.

Part 4 – Dirty for Life: making the good feelings last a lifetime

Easy tips on staying 'dirty for life' – reaching and maintaining your ideal healthy weight, plus great tips for keeping you and your microbiome happy, the dirty way!

Ready to get dirty?

I hope you're ready for the journey towards eating a balanced, delicious diet that will make you healthier *and* happier. I want you to feel *so* good on this diet that you want to stick to it for life. Dirty is the way forward . . . Let's tuck in!

Kate x

Health advice
and caution

**You should always consult a doctor
before making dietary changes.**

This book is written for information only and is not intended as medical advice, or as a substitute for medical advice, diagnosis or treatment.

Children, teenagers and pregnant and breastfeeding women shouldn't fast.

If you have a chronic condition or type 1 diabetes, it's particularly important that you consult your doctor, specialist or diabetes nurse before embarking on the Dirty Diet or making any significant change to your diet.

Many people with type 2 diabetes or metabolic syndrome have had success with intermittent fasting, but it's essential that you do this under supervision, especially if you are taking medication.

If you have any history of eating disorders, you should also consult a doctor or specialist before making any dietary change, including fasting.

Neither the author nor publisher or associates can be held responsible for any loss or claim resulting from the use or misuse of information and suggestions contained in this book, or for the failure to take medical advice.

Finally, never disregard professional medical advice or delay medical treatment because of something you have read in this book.

Note for those with allergies, intolerances, IBS or other digestive conditions

The Dirty Diet encourages a whole-food, diverse diet with plenty of fibre. If you have diagnosed allergies, or coeliac disease, do not disregard advice on foods you've been advised to avoid. Adapt accordingly and consult your dietitian to ensure your diet remains nutritionally balanced.

In addition, a rapid increase in the intake of dietary fibre can be challenging for people with IBS and other digestive conditions. **You should be aware of this, and introduce fibrous vegetables, pulses and wholegrains gradually, to allow your system and your gut microbes time to adapt.** If you have been advised to follow a low-FODMAP diet, the Dirty Diet may be possible following this with relevant personalised adaptation. Be sure to complete the low-FODMAP diet including the FODMAP reintroduction phase in full before starting the Dirty Diet, so that you are fully aware of the foods you can tolerate, and consult your dietitian first.

Part 1:
Dirty Diet Principles

The principles behind the Dirty Diet

I'd like to introduce you to your new way of life! It's one that's easy to adopt, wherever you live and whatever your circumstances or diet history.

In this chapter, I'll explain why the Dirty Diet works – and what you need to remember to make it work best for you. The foundations of the plan are science, research and real-life experiences. If you want to skip the science, you can go straight to Part 2 – you can start personalising the approach straight away – but it can really help to understand the *why* as you make positive changes. Our previous dirty dieters found it fascinating *and* highly motivating . . .

Despite the fact that I know our bodies contain bacteria, I didn't particularly want to think about that, and the idea of eating or drinking something that was full of 'friendly bacteria' freaked me out somewhat! I am now fascinated by the relationship between probiotics and prebiotics, and am consciously eating far more of the foods that my gut will love.

Kim, 53, housewife from Surrey, UK

I enjoyed the 'science' part of fasting, understanding the gut microbiome – it made a lot of sense to me and helped me understand the benefits of the diet from the start.

Holly, 38, HR consultant from Oxfordshire, UK

6 easy steps to Dirty Diet success

As I explained in the introduction, the Dirty Diet is easy to fit into your life. Here's a recap:

1. **On four or five days of the week – your 'Plenty Days' – you eat up to 1,800 calories per day.** The choices include easy recipes and ready-made options. Or use your own recipes and favourites!

2. **On two or three days – your 'Fast Days' – you scale back to 600–750 calories**, plus an extra portion of probiotic food like yogurt, kefir or pickle. Fill up on vegetables, with meat and fish options too. Fast Days help weight loss as well as mental/physical health.

3. You'll move towards **eating at least seven types of vegetable and fruit per day**: we'll show you how to work these into your meals, step by step.

4. **Nothing is banned:** we encourage variety, including full-fat dairy, grains, bread, meat, fish, coffee, alcohol and 'treats'. We encourage 'smart harvest' foods like cheese, yogurt, kefir and nuts or seeds (as well as dairy-free and nut-free alternatives).

5. **Bliss Moments** – your favourite foods – are included every week. Whether you love wine, cake or pizza, you

build those in every week, to help you love your food without the guilt.

6. **The only 'rule' is to cut out snacking** – and with our super-filling dishes, you won't need to eat between meals, or get cravings for the things your body doesn't need. In addition, we strongly recommend you reduce and, ideally, cut out artificial sweeteners.

To make the principles easier to remember, I've made them spell out the word DIRTY. Let's look at how and why they can each help transform your weight and health.

D is for **Diverse diet** – eating a wide range of fresh, whole ingredients. Plus the 'smart harvesting' tips that allow you to eat more and still lose weight.

I is for **Intermittent fasting** – limiting your calorie intake/ portion size on certain days to control weight and promote good health.

R is for **Restoring gut health** – promoting good digestion, immunity and mood by eating the right live foods (probiotics) and fibre (prebiotics).

T is for **Training yourself in healthy habits** – to encourage a long and active life.

Y is for **You** – how to customise the diet to suit your needs, tastes and goals.

D is for Diverse diet

Our first principle is prioritising variety in your diet: especially fresh vegetables, dairy, wholegrains, nuts and high-quality proteins.

A diverse, balanced diet matters because:

- Diversity means you're getting a wider spectrum of nutrients to support health and repair the body: it also ensures the diet includes lots of fibre.
- Not cutting out food groups means the diet is sustainable: unlike plans where food is banned, you can still enjoy the foods you love (though not in unlimited amounts!).
- Balance is important – overdoing a single ingredient, even supposed 'super-foods' like avocado or quinoa, means you miss out on other foods which have different benefits.
- Certain foods – like cheese, yogurt, nuts, oats, beans and even pasta and potatoes – can help you lose weight. We call this **'smart harvesting'** – read on to see how it works!

After years and years of hearing the old-fashioned views of what was 'fattening' and what wasn't, I was surprised how easily I dared give the hitherto-frowned-on foods a go, and how immediately it was obvious that this new information was revolutionary and . . . TRUE! Sourdough is now my non-guilty bread pleasure! I've also ditched the sweeteners after a double-figure number of years! Never thought THAT would be possible!

Helen B, 55, tutor from Devon, UK

Isn't weight all about the number of calories you eat?

People who've never struggled with their weight often say we get fat because we eat too much and don't move enough. On the surface this is true: you need to be consuming less energy than you're using to lose weight.

But there's another factor: *how* our bodies use the food that we're consuming. We all know people who eat very similar diets but end up at very different weights. Why is that?

- **Our genes:** in lean times, natural selection meant people who could maximise the energy from less food were likely to survive long enough to breed. So if you inherited those survival genes, you'll find weight loss harder.
- **Our environment:** where and how we live can make a big difference too, so even if you were born with genes that predispose you to weight gain, your behaviour and environment can stop that happening. Scientists are learning more all the time about how everything from our stress levels to upbringing and the air we breathe can affect how those genes behave.
- **Our gut bacteria:** each of us has a different balance of different bacteria. The balance can influence which nutrients are produced, and how much energy we absorb, as well as the health of our gut lining.

The research on how these factors interact has massive potential for human health, but the practical 'treatments' – like isolated strains of bacteria to address specific illnesses – are still quite limited.

However, the good news is there are delicious everyday foods that encourage weight loss: as part of the Dirty Diet, we suggest you make food choices that help with 'smart harvesting'. 'Smart harvesting' works in two main ways:

- Eating foods that **fill you up but lead to reduced fat absorption**.
- Eating foods that **temporarily increase calorie use**.

These are all tactics that Helen puts into practice with her clients who aren't losing weight despite a prolonged calorie deficit. The *number* of calories ˙you eat still matters, but being smart about the foods themselves can help our bodies too, as Helen explains:

> *Not all calories are equal. Some foods are better absorbed than others. When you consume almonds, for example, the amount of fat in your faeces goes up. This means we now know you do not absorb about 20 per cent of the calories in almonds. The same principle can be applied to other high-fibre whole unprocessed foods. In addition, calcium increases the fat in faeces, which explains why studies have shown a higher intake of cheese is related to lower body fat and body weight.*

---

* When we refer to calories in the book, we actually mean kilocalories. In Australia and New Zealand, kilojoules are used on packaging – one kilocalorie is 4.1 kilojoules.

I help clients focus on other ways to increase their body's
calorie consumption: increasing muscle mass through
resistance exercise, drinking green and white tea, eating spicy
food if they can tolerate it, drinking 500 ml of water before
each meal, and increasing calcium intake. These habits all
cause increased thermogenesis, which can be thought of as
'speeding up your metabolism'.

As we'll see in 'R is for Restoring gut health' (p. 52) – the foods we're recommending also influence our gut bacteria. Research suggests that if we eat a more varied and high-fibre diet, this leads to a more favourable microbiome, which does not harvest as many calories. If we follow an unvaried processed diet, the unbalanced microbe populations grab hold of every calorie they can get.

You'll be pleasantly surprised that our 'smart harvesting' foods are varied, and include many that dieters have traditionally been told are off limits, from full-fat dairy to pasta and potatoes.

'Smart harvest' strategy 1: Calcium-rich cheese and yogurt

Foods like cheese and yogurt – especially the full-fat versions – are often banned in weight loss diets. But they're actually great foods to include when you're trying to lose weight – so long as you keep the portion sizes to what we suggest in the plan and recipes! Here's why we love dairy:

1. The protein helps keep us fuller for longer so we don't seek out snacks;

2. The calcium speeds up your metabolism, so you burn calories faster;
3. And it also reduces the digestion of fat.

If you don't like dairy or are lactose intolerant, we suggest high calcium alternatives – like tofu, sardines or calcium-fortified soya or almond milk – but yogurt and cheese can still be an option for some people with an intolerance as the lactose content is severely reduced by fermentation.

> **Helen says:** *I focus on calcium intake as part of an effective weight loss strategy in my private clinic where I see fantastic results. Clients have often been put off dairy for fear of saturated fat, however three portions a day in the form of 200ml milk, a matchbox-size 30g of cheese and 125g pot of yogurt is often part of my recommended daily diet plan for healthy weight loss.*

Example recipes: Waldorf Muffins (p. 160), Greek Yogurt Fruit Sundae with Choc-Cherry Granola (p. 154).

'Smart harvest' strategy 2: Twice-cooked potatoes, pasta and rice, for resistant starch

Many diets avoid potatoes, rice and pasta because they can cause rapidly fluctuating blood sugar, which in turn can make us hungry and grumpy.

But simply heating potatoes, rice and pasta *and then allowing them to cool* changes their composition, and makes them better for us.

1. This cooking method creates resistant starches – a kind of starch that your gut microbes love, but that is less likely to lead to a sugar rush.
2. Dishes like a potato or rice salad, or a baked pasta dish that is later reheated, are better for you than when they're freshly cooked.

Helen says: When we think of fibre we often think of fruit, veg and wholegrains. But resistant starch is another type of fibre. It improves glycaemic control, which means it keeps your blood sugar levels better controlled, so is useful in managing diabetes. It also helps you feel full. One tactic I use with my clients to boost resistant starch is to save a portion of your carbs cooked at your evening meal for lunch the day after, think pasta, potato and rice salads.

Example recipes: Punchy New Potato Salad with Egg and Pea Shoots (p. 220), Chicken or Veggie Dirty Rice (pp. 206–208).

'Smart harvest' strategy 3: 'Swell' foods like oats, apples and barley that keep you feeling full

Foods like oats, barley and apples absorb water, which makes the food swell. This helps because:

1. The body takes longer to digest the food that's now larger in volume, so we feel fuller for longer. Insulin spikes are reduced, too.
2. These foods are loved by good gut microbes because they can digest them – the by-products of that digestive process help keep the gut lining healthy.

Helen says: *Oats are one of my favourite prebiotics – fuel for your microbes. When you eat oats, you're feeding your healthy bacteria and improving your microbiome, and encouraging all the health benefits. I recommend clients eat oats in some form daily.*

Example recipes: Overnight Power Oats with Fruit and Crunchy Nuts (p. 167), Barley Pot with Balsamic and Mustard Roast Winter Roots (p. 232).

'Smart harvest' strategy 4: nuts and seeds

Nuts and seeds are *so* good for us but appear high in calories. However, our bodies seem to absorb less energy from nuts and seeds than calorie charts suggest.

1. Nuts balance out the fats they contain with lots of fibre, so we don't absorb all the fat as they pass through the digestive system.
2. Walnuts and flaxseeds contain Omega 3 fatty acids, which help to regulate and improve blood sugar and fat metabolism.
3. They're satisfying and tasty due to the fat, protein and fibre content so we don't feel hungry as quickly.

Helen says: *From eating nuts daily as part of the Mediterranean diet to eating a handful of almonds a day as part of the cholesterol-targeting Portfolio diet, nuts have consistently been shown to improve health. Enjoy your nuts with the skin on to maximise fibre intake and the health benefits they provide.*

Example recipes: Beef, Mushroom and Cashew Stir Fry (p. 228), Quick-as-a-Flash Cauliflower and Broccoli Tabbouleh (p. 187).

Bonus smart harvest ingredient: Mushrooms

Fungi pack a punch – one year-long study showed that a group of obese people who ate mushrooms instead of red meat lost weight and inches from the waist, improved their blood pressure and other blood test results. They also maintained the weight loss. Including more mushrooms in *your* diet helps because:

1. They're a fantastic source of plant-based protein – with very low calories.
2. The protein makes them filling – one study showed people who had mushrooms at breakfast ate less during the day than those who chose meat – and they can also help to regulate blood sugar.

Helen says: *There is a wealth of published scientific research on mushrooms which has revealed them to be anti-oxidative, immune-enhancing, anti-inflammatory and prebiotic. All these properties mean they have been shown to help reduce hypertension, blood sugar levels in diabetics, obesity and cholesterol. They are also being studied for their potential to treat cancer and Alzheimer's. In addition, they are a great dietary source of vitamin D – if you expose them to direct sunlight 1–2 hours before cooking, this boosts their vitamin D content further.*

Example recipes: Mushroom and Black Bean Koftas (p. 238), Mushroom and Tofu Stroganoff (p. 209).

Smarter, fuller, slimmer

No single food is magic in itself – and all food adds calories to your diet, so you need to be portion-aware. But including these ingredients in your diet can improve your health and weight loss speed. Plus, in line with Dirty Diet principles, they taste amazing . . .

THE DIRTY DIET TAKEOUT: D is for a Diverse diet

- A diverse, balanced diet helps you get all the varied nutrients you need.
- It also reduces feelings of deprivation or cravings because nothing is banned.
- Certain foods – including dairy, nuts, twice-cooked starch and other fibres – provide extra benefits to help you lose weight.

THE DIRTY DIET IN ACTION
'A diverse diet – including wine and cheese –
that's worth celebrating'

Kim, 53, housewife from Surrey, UK

After 28 days: 9lbs (4kg) lost, 23.6 BMI (down from 25.2), fewer cravings, better gut health, and improved menopausal symptoms.

Kim says: I love cheese and I love wine, and the prospect of a way of eating that really celebrates good food of the sort that is often 'forbidden' was wonderful. I have finally bought size 10 jeans and they fit!

I haven't worn a size 10 since I was in my early 20s – so for 30 years! I now have a waist again and can wear fitted clothes and feel they look good after years of buying oversized baggy clothes to hide my shape. I am getting so many compliments from friends and acquaintances, and I have also been told that I am looking younger.

I am thrilled with the changes to my body, but more importantly with the changes to my diet and the way that I have begun to understand how my body reacts to different foods. Rather than just feeling slimmer and lighter, I am eating far more healthily than I was before, and I feel so much better for the variety and diversity of the foods I am eating. I have discovered kefir which I now love, and have also discovered a passion for Greek yogurt, when previously the only yogurts I would ever have eaten were the highly flavoured low-calorie fat-free versions. I am now fascinated by the relationship between probiotics and prebiotics and am consciously eating far more of the foods that my gut will love. I love cheese but had begun to see it as a bit of a 'danger' food. Now I incorporate it into my diet and it is far less of a trigger.

I have spent much of my adult life on a diet. I have tried Weight Watchers, the F-plan, the Atkins diet, the cabbage soup diet, several other popular 'fad' diets, and the 5:2 diet. On many of the above I lost weight very quickly but often felt unwell, could not sustain weight loss and ended up putting more back on. I had already lost 5 stone following Kate's 5:2 books. 5:2 was very good for me in terms of weight loss, but the big difference with the Dirty Diet is that I have begun to think about health, not just weight loss, and am making far better choices about what I eat, both on Fast Days and on Plenty Days. I feel the Dirty Diet is something I will now live with for life – I don't want to lose any more weight, but I do want to maintain my current weight and I want to keep this healthier way of life for good.

Health changes: It has improved my gut health, as I used to get heartburn sometimes and also suffered with a fair amount of diarrhoea and 'looseness' which has totally cleared up now. I am also far more 'regular' than I have been for years, and just feel as if my whole system is better.

Insomnia has been an increasing problem over the past year or so, possibly related to the perimenopause, but had become almost intolerable. Since being on the Dirty Diet my sleep patterns are much better. My mood and self-esteem were also low before the Dirty Diet, both of which have improved significantly. I think the choice of food is what has improved my mood, and my perimenopausal symptoms have improved. I had resorted to using gel pillows to cool my body down at night because I was overheating so badly at times, and have hardly used them since being on the Dirty Diet.

Top tips: Other people's testimonies have been a real help – read these for motivation. Also, don't feel you have to read everything in one go. Get started, then go back to the principles a little at a time: after just four weeks I feel I have a much better understanding of nutrition and how the body processes different foods. I feel I know my own body better and am making much better choices.

I is for Intermittent fasting

Intermittent fasting (IF) means scheduling days when you eat lower-calorie meals, or extending the times where you don't eat at all. It's a brilliantly simple strategy that:

- helps you lose weight;
- teaches you to understand your appetite better (and avoid over-eating in future);
- can benefit gut health;
- allows your body to repair itself.

IF has changed my life and my attitude to food, as it has for hundreds of thousands of other people. It's been way easier than I could have expected, and has been the most sustainable food strategy I've ever started. I do it every week, over five years after I began. And I had to include it as central to the Dirty Diet because it's so simple and powerful.

How does the Dirty Diet incorporate intermittent fasting?

The most popular form of IF has been 5:2 – two days of cutting back, five eating normally. But in the Dirty Diet, we're adding flexibility to the Fast Days, so you could do three days a week instead of two, to speed up results. We encourage you to build meals around vegetables, because they're filling and low-calorie. You can either go meat-free, or include leaner proteins like chicken breast fillets and white fish.

> I have tried Slimming World and Weight Watchers in the past, but I find fasting works better as it teaches you about when you are actually hungry, and about only eating when you need to, not eating because you feel you have to. Now I feel in control, I sleep much better, and I don't feel so bloated.
>
> Alex, 34, resuscitation officer, Hampshire, UK

The simplest strategy for coping with a world full of food

Conventional dieting is hard. We're bombarded with advertising for high-energy processed food, which in itself has been engineered to be as irresistible as possible.

But intermittent fasting gives us a completely flexible framework to help us eat better.

- Choosing to cut right back on two to three days a week can be much easier than having to resist all high-energy foods all the time.

- Overall calorie reduction promotes weight loss – fasting on two or three days creates a calorie deficit which our body will deal with by using fat reserves for energy.
- Gaps between eating encourage that fat-burning to happen.
- Fasting teaches you that allowing yourself to feel temporarily hungry isn't scary or dangerous, but is a useful signal that helps you avoid over-eating at other times.

As someone who loves her food, I really wasn't sure when I started my first Fast Day whether I'd have the willpower to avoid eating. But I found that having the right attitude, and understanding the health benefits, made it easy. It was a choice I was making for my own body. And feeling a bit hungry isn't a big deal – I realised soon that I could ignore those signals and they'd go away – and I wasn't doing myself any harm. In fact, it was the opposite.

The power of fasting for health

Fasting helps the body's immune and digestive systems heal and regenerate: in other words, it helps the body to **repair itself.**

The body is brilliant at multitasking. But like us, it works better when it doesn't have quite as much to deal with. Think of how hard it is to watch TV, look after the kids, *and* read this book at the same time? Now imagine turning off the TV and sending the kids to bed, and being able to read undistracted and uninterrupted.

Digestion is a demanding process for the body, but when you increase the periods of time between eating it can focus on other things that tend to get neglected.

In addition, **fasting stresses the body in a positive way**. It's similar to exercise in this way: when you go for a jog or lift some weights, you're putting your heart, lungs and muscles under stress, but your body responds by getting stronger and fitter. Fasting does this too – sensing a lack of food, the body begins to 'tune up' the cells to help them act more efficiently.

Our bodies are made up of around 30 trillion cells (give or take 7 trillion!), which control everything from basic functions like breathing, to advanced mental functions like problem-solving or dealing with emotions. But cells divide multiple times, and whenever they do, they risk malfunctioning, which can cause diseases, including cancer.

When the body is in a fasting state, it **identifies malfunctioning cells and either repairs them or, if necessary, kills them off** and allows them to be recycled. This 'programmed cell death' is protective against cancer.

Another key factor in why we develop disease is **inflammation – an immune response to injury or illness**. If you're hurt or ill, your body sends specialist cells and activates chemicals to isolate the danger. The first sign is often heat or swelling, because blood flow increases to move the 'special forces' into place. If the system works, the attacker is eliminated, the affected cells die, and the immune system and blood flow return to normal.

But when the body doesn't call off the special forces – either because it's still under attack or the immune system mistakenly thinks it is – **inflammation becomes damaging**. Imagine your internal organs and circulatory system constantly swollen and inflamed, and you begin to understand why. It's associated with many diseases, including diabetes, heart disease, cancer, auto-immune conditions such as rheumatoid arthritis, and dementia.

The same cell 'tune-up' process can reduce inflammation too: the exact processes are only just becoming understood, but it's one of the reasons fasting may have greater health benefits than those that result from simply losing weight.

So what does this all achieve? The body of research into intermittent fasting is growing all the time, but animal and human studies have shown:

- **Improved insulin response:** Longer gaps between meals mean insulin levels have a chance to drop, allowing us to burn body fat rather than store more for energy. Our blood sugar can thus fall to healthier levels and our body's response to insulin can also improve, reducing our chances of developing type 2 diabetes.
- **Short-term fasting can speed up metabolism**, the rate at which we use energy – which helps us lose weight or maintain a healthy weight. It has also been shown to help us lose a better ratio of fat to muscle than conventional very-low-calorie diets.
- **Boosts focus:** Concentration can be improved by short-term fasting, as certain proteins and hormones that influence focus, memory and mood are activated. On an evolutionary level, the smarter and more resourceful humans were in times of famine, the higher their chances of survival.
- **Reduced 'markers'** of inflammation in blood tests – which may then lead to lower incidence of cardiovascular disease and degenerative brain conditions (for example, in studies

involving mice and rats, fasting helped delay the onset
and decrease symptoms in those genetically susceptible to
degenerative brain conditions).

- **May improve life expectancy:** In some animal studies,
  a controlled, calorie-restricted diet has been shown to
  increase longevity and also health into old age. It's harder
  for humans to maintain calorie restriction, but intermittent
  fasting can be a more acceptable way to reduce calorie
  intake long term.
- **Fasting – together with probiotics – can increase the
  diversity of your gut microbiome** – see R is for Restoring
  gut health (p. 52) for more on why this is positive. Fasting
  was shown to boost one strain in particular – Akkermansia
  – which keeps the walls of the large intestine healthy.

A word about eating between meals and the snacking myth

Many people who hear about intermittent fasting for the first
time are surprised – they've heard some nutritionists say that
eating small, regular meals helps boost metabolism (the process
of using energy).

In addition, for decades now, food manufacturers have urged
us to snack between meals – as though feeling peckish is the
worst thing in the world. But they're not thinking of *your* health
– it's more that the more food they sell, the bigger their profits.

For most of us, eating between meals is a terrible idea!

But what about the caveman, you might say? He ate when
he could – a few berries here and a nut there. Compare that to
what *we* do:

- Most modern snacks are high in calories.
- We're not having to walk long distances to find them.
- Although metabolism is boosted after eating, that boost is rarely enough to cancel out the extra calories you're taking in.
- Biologically, it's bad for us too – especially if we want to stay a healthy weight. The hormone insulin goes to work after we've eaten, to control blood sugar and store excess energy as fat. Critically, when insulin is at work in the body, we can't burn fat – which is what we want to do to lose weight.

Taking intermittent fasting further: 16:8

A close cousin of 5:2 is 'time-limited eating' – the most popular form is called '16:8'. This is where you only eat during set time 'windows', and avoid food the rest of the time. With 16:8, you're aiming for an 8-hour period of eating, and 'fasting' the rest of the time. So you might eat brunch at 10.30 a.m., lunch at 2 p.m. and dinner no later than 6 p.m. The rest of the time, you can still drink fluids, but ideally calorie-free ones: water, black coffee, black tea, herbal teas.

You don't necessarily have to reduce calories during the eating window itself, though often this happens naturally as fewer meals are consumed, leading to weight loss. And it's thought that these windows could offer many of the health advantages of 5:2 from p. 39. You could also adapt the window e.g. adopt a 14:10 approach. What works best varies from person to person, so do experiment if you think it could be a useful part of your routine.

Intermittent fasting for beginners: a quick guide to your Fast Days

I love my Fast Days with a passion! But if you've never tried intermittent fasting before, here is a quick guide to getting started.

What counts as a Fast Day?

A Fast Day lasts from the last meal the previous day until breakfast the day after. For example:

Sunday: Eat dinner/last meal of the day at normal time, e.g. 7 p.m.

Monday: Fast Day – eat 500–650 calories (or less), over no more than three meals

Tuesday: Eat breakfast/first meal of the day at your normal time, e.g. 8 a.m.

Which days should I choose?

Separate your Fast Days at first. For example, fast on Monday and Wednesday, or Tuesday and Thursday. It's easier to stick to your limit when you know that tomorrow you can eat what you like. Once you're used to fasting, you can do a 'back to back', i.e. two days in succession.

For your first fasts, choose days when you're busy but not under serious work or family pressure. You can change days each week to suit your diary.

When should I eat on Fast Days? And how often?

The Speedy Plan suggests two meals, and the Steady Plan three smaller ones. Leaving longer gaps between eating, or only eating one or two meals, may increase the health benefits of fasting.

Many 5:2 dieters, including me, began by eating three very small meals, but now skip breakfast or lunch and either eat twice or just once instead. Some of us definitely find that the later we leave it to eat, the less hungry we feel.

Some people find water fasts/juice fasts easier. Personally, I prefer to eat solid food, and you should remember that fruit-based juices are high in sugar and sometimes calories. Also, eating fruits or vegetables whole means they're digested more slowly, which staves off hunger pangs for longer. But juice fasts should be safe for one day at a time if you're in good health and not taking medication. Check with your doctor if you have any concerns at all.

Practical tips

Here are some tips to help you adapt, and you can find many more on my YouTube channel: http://bit.ly/1t8aBtr

- **Drink plenty of water, black coffee, tea or low-cal herbal teas.** Milk can affect insulin levels but can still be included in the fast. Diet drinks also may affect insulin and gut bacteria in unhelpful ways so are best avoided.
- **Distract yourself**. Hunger tends to come in waves, so do things that take your mind off it until it subsides. Make yourself a drink, visit the Facebook group, phone a friend

or read a book. The Dirty Diet support group on Facebook is a closed group, so posts won't be visible to friends on your timeline.

- **Move more.** Many of us go for a run or to the gym on a Fast Day with no difference in stamina or performance. Just be careful and listen to your body the first couple of times, taking a break if need be, and make sure you stay hydrated. And no, you can't 'earn' extra calories on a Fast Day, but you will feel virtuous afterwards.
- **Don't panic if you're peckish.** Remember that it's positive to **relearn what appetite feels like**, and how smaller meals than we're used to can still be satisfying.
- **Celebrate food.** When you *do* eat, make an occasion of it if possible. Lay the table, use pretty plates, pour yourself some water and add a slice of lemon, play relaxing music. And savour every bite . . . eating this way is more satisfying to the senses!
- Finally, remember the 5:2 catchphrase: **'Tomorrow you can eat what you like.'** Though most of us find the next day we're not that hungry!

Fasting trouble-shooter

Fasting can help our health by placing us under good stress, just as exercise does. But like starting to run or lift weights, your Fast Days can feel strange at first. Our daily lives are often built around mealtimes, so changing that routine feels odd initially. Plus, many of us have forgotten how it feels to be hungry!

Most people get through their first Fast Days with no unwelcome changes. However, there are a few sensations that you might experience, all of which can be managed.

- **Feeling cold** – This is common in winter, partly because your body generates more heat when it's digesting food. Try drinking hot drinks and wearing extra layers.
- **Headaches** – These are common when making any dietary change due to dehydration and/or changes to blood sugar. This should settle over time, but drinking plenty of water, or taking a mild painkiller, will help.
- **Irritability** – You may feel grumpy at first: that's low blood sugar again. Try to build in a non-food treat to look forward to: a long hot bath, a hand massage, or perhaps your favourite TV show.
- **Digestive changes** – As you're not eating as much you may not need to open your bowels as often, or you may find that the next day your digestion is slower (or faster) than normal. Most people find that their digestion settles as they adapt to the new way of eating.
- **Feeling light-headed** – This is much less common, but having a small snack ready (maybe something from the Side dishes section on p. 254) can help. If you feel very unwell, eat normally and take medical advice before trying a second fast.

THE DIRTY DIET TAKEOUT:
I is for Intermittent fasting

- Fasting is a strategy to help us reach and stay a healthy weight.
- It can also help the body repair itself and therefore prevent disease.
- In addition, fasting may increase the diversity of good bacteria in the gut, including one strain that helps the lining stay healthy.
- Increasing the time between eating – and cutting out snacking – helps us understand our appetite and the emotional factors that can also make us want to eat.

THE DIRTY DIET IN ACTION
'Intermittent fasting gives you freedom'

Sarah, 42, deputy principal, Perth, Australia

After 28 days: lost 12lbs (5.5kg), 32.8 BMI (down from 34.8), sleeping well, feeling liberated.

Sarah says: I sleep more soundly, feel happier, and have more energy – I even got on my eight-year-old daughter's scooter this afternoon!

I have tried so many other diets, and in the last couple of years I have felt lost: knowing that I need to lose weight to be around for my eight-year-old daughter, knowing that my eating was killing me, but feeling so overwhelmed by all the different diets. Should I eat clean, should I eat Paleo, or do low-carb/high-fat? I was wondering if surgery was the only way, but knowing that could also kill me, and wishing every day I could go to any shop to buy clothes. My weight was causing me unhappiness and bringing me down every day, making me look so much older than my age . . . Now I feel liberated, I feel in control of my eating and I've had compliments already, especially with regards to my skin. My clothes feel better (I need to look for new work trousers as they are getting loose!) and I feel I've been given a chance to succeed at what I have wanted for so long.

Since starting the Dirty Diet I have been eating *such* delicious, healthy food. I have had NO takeaways, and after a few days I gave up Diet Cokes and other soft drinks, as that went hand in hand with my commitment to the Dirty Diet. Overall it has been an easy diet and I love the element of calorie counting. This gives me the control I need but also the accountability for everything I eat. My eating habits have changed dramatically: I learned that hunger was just another feeling, and it didn't mean I had to stuff something in my mouth every time I felt hungry – I could work through it. As for what I do eat, the Dirty Diet has helped me taste food again and has given me so many ideas – it's exactly what I needed!

Top tips: Introduce new foods slowly – don't overwhelm yourself. Don't be afraid of the Fast Days: use them to have control. And embrace the calorie counting; you'll be shocked how many calories you were probably consuming before the Dirty Diet!

R is for Restoring gut health

Our guts – in fact, our entire digestive system – matter more than we ever imagined. Without digestion, there is no fuel for our bodies. And without fuel, we can't function.

Yet modern life – including processed foods, antibiotics, disordered eating and lack of fibre – can play havoc with a healthy digestive system. That's why restoring gut health is a priority. The good news is it's easy to improve by eating the right live foods (probiotics) and fibre (prebiotics).

The even better news? A healthy gut can help everything from your mood to your immune system – and your weight, of course.

Once I'd committed to this way of eating I found myself learning why gut bacteria are my friends! I now think about what I am eating so that I can maximise my gut health. The result is that not only do I feel better and have more energy, but I am sleeping better and I have lost inches and lost weight, despite the fact that I am eating more – what a result!

Kim

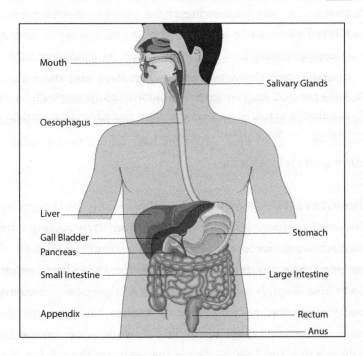

The wonderful world of your microbiome

You have an organ no one even knew existed 10 years ago. Certainly, there are no drawings of it in school biology textbooks. Yet it influences weight control, mental health, diabetes, immunity, allergies, asthma, digestion, vitamin and hormone production and countless other processes that keep us alive.

It's the gut microbiome, and it's not like any other organ – because it's composed of trillions of tiny bacteria and other lifeforms that live inside our lower intestine. Their combined genetic material interacts with ours, to work for us, or against us: and many of medicine's biggest mysteries may be on their way to being solved as scientists discover more about how they function. The first sequencing of the human microbiome was published as recently as 2012: the knowledge we're already gaining is changing how we look at ourselves fundamentally.

Microbes are present almost everywhere on, and in, our bodies: the make-up of each 'colony' varies dramatically, with different bacteria existing on our teeth, under our arms, in our noses, even in our eyes. And they have a huge part to play in our health and wellbeing.

The ecosystem in your gut

The colony in your large intestine is currently attracting most interest from doctors and researchers. The 'microbiome' – meaning the ecosystem these microbes form together – weighs up to 5lbs (3kg). It influences so many of the body's functions, and treatments are already being trialled to target the gut bacteria to treat a range of conditions, while more commercial supplements and 'live' foods are appearing on the market. You can even have your microbiome 'tested' – at a price.

There's a lot still to discover, but we do know that our gut microbiome appreciates a diverse diet with loads of plant-based and high-fibre food – exactly what we're recommending in the Dirty Diet. We'll give lots of practical tips later – but for now, let's look at the science.

Why is it so important to look after our friendly microbes? Because we need them to look after us back . . .

Dirty little helpers

All kids are taught to avoid 'filthy germs' and anything that looks 'dirty'. But that's a very one-sided view of the microbes that have been evolving alongside us for millennia.

Developments in DNA sequencing mean we can now count and identify the microbes through genetic testing of human faeces, and begin to understand the microbes' own history and their functions. What we've discovered already has completely changed how we see many aspects of health and medicine. Incredibly, solutions to many chronic health concerns – from obesity to diabetes, degenerative brain disease to asthma – could lie in our own personal colonies. Some of these bacteria benefit us in astonishing ways – producing hormones, vitamins and other chemicals that help our bodies function well, digesting food, and helping create a robust immune system.

But other hostile or 'pathogenic' bacteria can make us more vulnerable to chronic diseases, weight gain and even depression or anxiety: if they get out of balance, we feel their effects.

Gut health = the answer to weight loss, mood and health puzzles?

When I began to read research about the body's bacteria influencing weight, health and mood, it seemed far-fetched. But the more I read, the more I felt the same excitement as those many scientists and doctors who believe the microbiome could be the missing link.

But what is it the microbes are doing? To understand that, let's take a speedy tour of our digestive system. If you're a bit squeamish, don't read this before eating!

The big tube

Medics often describe the digestive system as a big tube – the mouth at one end, taking the food in, and your anus at the other end, getting rid of the waste products, once your body has removed all the nutrients and water it can use.

The process of digesting our food starts before we've even taken a bite. You know how even thinking of your favourite meal makes your mouth water? Saliva contains enzymes that start the process of turning food into fuel as we chew. The process continues when chewed food travels down the oesophagus into the highly acidic environment in our stomach. The stomach churns the food – breaking down proteins, the building blocks that make and repair cells.

Next comes the small intestine, where juices produced by the liver and pancreas help make fats, vitamins and minerals in food usable by your body. Those nutrients head towards the liver, while the waste products go towards the gut or large intestine: this is where your microbiome lives. As the food and the gas created by digestion travel, you get a familiar rumbling known as borborygmus (the technical term for gurgling and Helen's favourite word!).

Digestion, production, protection: what the good bacteria are up to in our guts

By the time food reaches your large intestine, the body has done what it can to break down your meal. Now it's the turn of the bacteria, and nine other kinds of microbes, to get busy with the leftovers *we* can't use. So what do they do? We're only just discovering their many functions, but so far we know the following.

Your good microbes can . . .	Why this matters . . .
MAKE vitamins, including B12, folate, biotin and thiamine. Bifidobacterium strains are especially good at producing B vitamins.	These vitamins help repair our DNA, promote development of a baby in the womb, influence cell growth, and protect the brain and nervous system.
HELP the gut work effectively.	Good bacteria help faeces move through the gut at the right pace.
REINFORCE the gut lining by producing short-chain fatty acids (SCFAs) including: - Acetate - Propionate - Butyrate	These acids, especially butyrate, provide fuel for the cells that line the gut, helping to produce mucus that strengthens the gut wall. This prevents toxins in the gut from entering the rest of the body, which is what occurs with a 'leaky gut'. SCFAs have been shown to protect against colon cancer.
REDUCE inflammation elsewhere in the body.	SCFAs help to reduce inflammation in the body, which is linked to cancer, cardiovascular disease and many other conditions.
TEACH your immune system how to recognise real danger (and ignore minor threats).	The SCFAs also help to regulate the production of immune cells – these help the body tell the difference between damaging invaders and minor threats, or even our own cells. Autoimmune diseases like type 1 diabetes and thyroid conditions are caused when the immune system gets it wrong, and attacks vital organs like the pancreas or thyroid gland.

STOP dangerous microbes taking over.	The right balance of beneficial bacteria stops pathogens getting out of control.
MAKE hormones and neurochemicals which influence the brain and nervous system. Lactobacillus strains are important in the production of these.	The microbes are particularly important in producing 90% of the body's serotonin, known to play a vital role in depression and anxiety.
ACT directly on the nervous system through the 'gut–brain axis' via the vagus nerve.	This can send signals which directly affect the brain and nervous system, influencing memory, mood, sleep, stress and many other mental functions. Some gut microbes can influence behaviour. For example, the toxoplasma gondii parasite has been shown to alter both rodent and human behaviour, making us less risk-averse and even having a part to play in some mental illnesses. Often these illnesses are accompanied with digestive problems.
HARVEST energy and regulate fat storage.	A diverse, balanced microbiome can ensure nutrients are harvested but weight stays healthy.

Overall, it's a pretty astonishing list – and when you consider that the research on the microbiome is relatively new, you begin to see the potential for diagnosis and treatment of human diseases and disorders. But what does it mean for you personally?

The life story of YOUR microbiome

You were born without any microbes in your gut – what happened to you after that has influenced which ones live there now. Including:

- How you were born: vaginal birth introduces a different set of microbes to those a new baby receives during a Caesarean section;
- How many courses of antibiotics you were given for childhood infections;
- What you were fed and where you live;
- Even the people and/or animals you live with right now influence your microbiome.

So how could what's happening in your gut be affecting your whole body? We're only just starting to piece things together. But, as an example, farmers know that feeding livestock low levels of antibiotics doesn't only serve to protect them from infection – it also means they put on more weight than animals that don't receive constant doses. In humans, the rise in childhood and adult obesity has coincided with the widespread use of antibiotics. The suggestion is that a less diverse microbiome could be a factor.

In particular, the rises in obesity, allergies and auto-immune conditions since the 1940s have coincided with the development of antibiotics, which wipe out a lot of the 'good guys' at the same time as eliminating the disease-carrying bacteria we were *trying* to target. If you've ever had diarrhoea after a course of antibiotics, you'll know these medications can have unintended, but short-term, consequences: our balance usually restores itself in time. Repeated courses of antibiotics can be much more harmful.

Changes to the microbiome may also hold the key to understanding the dramatic increase in the number of children with allergic conditions, from asthma to potentially fatal peanut allergies. And studies of the microbiomes of children with autistic spectrum disorder also show they have significant differences to those in children who don't have it. Whether these are cause or effect, we don't yet know.

Let's take a quick tour of some areas that might affect you:

The weight factor

- The guts of people who are obese contain different microbes to those who aren't. The bacteria producing SCFAs I mentioned in the table are important. People of normal weight tend to have more of these, so the bacteria then generate more SCFAs, with all the benefits this brings. Recent research suggests a diverse gut microbiome is more about a diverse, healthy diet than what a person actually weighs – but research on the precise mechanisms is underway.
- Experiments show that transplanting gut contents – that's poo to you and me – can lead to weight loss or gain, according to the microbes of the donor. In one case, a 32-year-old woman being treated for an infection put on 33 pounds after receiving a transplant from her 16-year-old daughter, who also became obese. But other studies have shown that when poo is transplanted from a person

of normal weight into the gut of an overweight person or one with type 2 diabetes, many do lose weight or see an improved response to insulin. Much more work is needed to isolate the microbes involved.

- These 'poo transplants' are also being used for ulcerative colitis, irritable bowel syndrome, and the notoriously difficult to treat bacterial gut infection, Clostridium difficile (which can affect those already in poor health, especially in hospitals).

The disease factor

- 'Abnormal' or untypical microbiomes have been shown in people suffering from a whole range of diseases, including inflammatory bowel disease, psoriasis, dermatitis, auto-immune diseases, type 2 diabetes, Parkinson's disease, multiple sclerosis, chronic fatigue syndrome and other conditions.
- There may also be a connection between Alzheimer's, as certain gut bacteria can produce the plaques or lumps that are seen in the brain as the disease develops.
- We can't yet pinpoint which bacteria may play a role – and whether they play a part in causing the conditions, or are simply present as a side-effect of a disease that's already present.

The mental health factor

- Depression, anxiety and mood disorders have been linked to how the gut bacteria affect what's known as the gut–brain axis. That's the connection between the brain and the nerve cells in the lining of the gut. There is a constant stream of messages going back and forth, most coming from the gut to the brain. Experts have called the digestive system 'the second brain' because it's so important to our mental function and our behaviour.

- The microbiome is the third element in the chain of command. Chemicals produced by the bacteria can affect our actions and thoughts both positively and negatively.
- Research shows differences in the human gut microbiome of people with a range of mental health conditions, including anxiety, obsessive compulsive disorders, alcoholism and anorexia nervosa.
- Studies have shown positive results from probiotics in a range of patients, from women suffering from stress and depression to hospital patients suffering from hard-to-treat digestive bugs worsened by constant use of antibiotics.

What should I do now?

I'm definitely **not** suggesting any DIY transplantation. And if you suspect your gut microbes might have been affected by life events, please don't obsess about that; antibiotics and Caesarean births are lifesavers.

The good news is your microbiome can be improved through diet. So even if yours isn't as balanced or diverse as it could be, the Dirty Diet will help you change that for the good. And it doesn't have to be expensive.

Restoring and supporting your microbiome with the Dirty Diet

You can make changes to your microbiome very quickly by altering your diet. It's been shown that the balance can shift within 24 hours when a dramatic change is made, like switching from a meat-based diet to a plant-based one, or vice versa. Those changes are short-lived, however; so making sustainable changes to your diet has to be the answer.

Foods your gut microbes love

These foods can all promote a healthier balance:

- **Non-digestible carbs/fibre:** these are vital to good gut health because the microbes ferment these, producing beneficial short-chain fatty acids (SCFAs). Fibre-rich foods that can help include beans, wheat, raw oats, chicory root (used to produce inulin powder, a health supplement), resistant starches like cooked-then-cooled potatoes, pasta and rice – we include them in the Dirty Diet meal plans and recipes for this reason.
- **Probiotics** like fermented milk (e.g. yogurt and a delicious drink called kefir which we will talk a lot about in this book), sour veggie pickles, and some non-dairy alternatives increase the range of good bacteria and limit the less beneficial ones. They also improve digestion generally, cholesterol and insulin sensitivity – a factor in type 2 diabetes. A probiotic supplement can also help if you don't like or can't tolerate dairy or ferments (see p. 320 for guidance).

63

- **Polyphenols** – these often highly coloured compounds are found in fruit, vegetables, seeds, cocoa, black and especially green tea, as well as red wine – they improve gut diversity, and numbers of harmful bacteria can also be reduced by powerful polyphenols in fruit skin.
- **Protein:** vegetable proteins (from all kinds of legumes/ beans and peas) promote the production of the healthy SCFAs better than animal proteins. High-animal-protein diets are not associated with the same diversity, perhaps because they also tend to be higher in fat. High-animal-protein diets also increase IGF-1, which can be associated with faster development of cancer and inflammation.
- **Fat:** monounsaturated fats – like olive oil and some fish oils – increase levels of good bacteria, including Bifidobacteria and Akkermansia muciniphila. Diets very high in animal fats are associated with less diversity and lower butyrate/ SCFA levels.
- **Carbohydrates:** digestible carbs – i.e. starches and sugars – are associated with a higher level of Bifidobacteria.

Foods and habits that *don't* benefit your gut microbes

As with the other research, it's early days, but the following may affect gut diversity:

- **Gluten-free diets.** Cutting out gluten has been shown to lower populations of healthy Bifidobacterium and Lactobacillus. Obviously for those with coeliac disease, this is unavoidable – and other wholegrains may help – but it's a good reason to maintain diversity for those without coeliac disease or diagnosed intolerances.

- **High-protein, low-carb diets.** This type of diet can also reduce diversity. This shouldn't be a surprise – most low-carb diets, including the Paleo approach, severely restrict or ban wholegrains. Yet as we've seen, these are a brilliant fuel source for your gut bacteria. For me, it makes no sense at all to remove something that's enjoyable for me and my microbes.

- **Artificial sweeteners.** These appear to be worse for the gut than natural sugars like fructose and lactose. This is the reason I've all but eliminated artificial sweeteners – including all low-cal and diet drinks – from my diet and now use sugar, honey, maple syrup or fruit when some sweetness really is needed in a dish. Try to eliminate or at least cut down.

- **Emulsifiers.** These additives are used to make foods like ice-cream and mayonnaise bind, to create an appealing mouth-feel/texture. But they've been shown to change the gut balance in mice. Foods that are naturally emulsified by combining fat with protein e.g. home-made mayo, may not have the same effect.

Probiotics vs prebiotics

These two words cause confusion but they're very different, though both are important for improved gut health.

Probiotics are 'live' foods or supplements containing good bacteria: by taking them, you're aiming to introduce new colonies or populations of the beneficial microbes into your gut. These include:

- Fermented plain dairy including Greek yogurt, kefir and some of the cultured drinks and yogurts branded as probiotic e.g. Yakult, Actimel and Activia. Other traditional drinks include amasi (a Zulu drink) and laban, found in the Middle East.
- Non-dairy alternatives like coconut kefir (though if you have a lactose intolerance, you **may** still be able to consume both Greek yogurt and dairy kefir, as much of the lactose has been digested by the beneficial bacteria: people vary in their tolerance of fermented milk products).
- Some cheese – the smellier and stronger it is, the more likely it contains live bacteria. Blue cheese is one where you even can see the bacterial activity!
- Sour vegetable pickles, including sauerkraut and kimchi, which have not been heat-treated.
- Supplements – either in capsule or powder form – of specific strains or a mix of different beneficial bacteria (see p. 320 for instructions on what to look for).

Prebiotics are types of dietary fibre that we can't fully digest but which your good bacteria love: by eating foods containing these special types of fibre, or taking a supplement, you're giving the microbes fuel that they turn into the vitamins, SCFAs and other products we want to encourage. You're also creating an environment that encourages more of the good bacteria to stick around in your gut. Prebiotics include:

- Inulin and fructooligosaccharides (FOS), (found in onions, garlic, asparagus, bananas, chicory root and Jerusalem artichokes).
- Others include pectin (found in apples), beta-glucans (found in oats and other water-loving grains) and resistant starch (found in cooked-then-cooled starchy foods like potato and rice).
- Supplements, e.g. inulin powder from chicory root. These can be really powerful and health-giving – see p. 323 for more information.
- Synthetically produced prebiotics added to food.

Don't worry about remembering all the details, though. The Dirty Diet encourages adding more pre- and probiotics to your meals without fuss!

The Dirty Diet takeout:
R is for Restoring your microbiome

- A balanced gut microbiome is key to good mental and physical health.
- The microbiome can be altered through a healthy diet.
- The Dirty Diet includes probiotics, prebiotics and other whole ingredients that promote great gut health and keep your trillions of microbes happy.

THE DIRTY DIET IN ACTION
'Better gut health helps your skin glow
and your mood soar'

Jane, 53, nurse from Dubai

After 28 days: lost 9lbs (4kg), 22.1 BMI (down from 23.15), better gut health and mood, acne improved.

Jane says: I was already a healthy BMI but I wanted to try the Dirty Diet to achieve some weight loss and a flatter stomach – and I'm glad I did! I only recently began to get a spare tyre and thought it was with me for ever post-menopause, but my work colleague says my stomach has gone – and my husband says my bum's smaller!

My acne rosacea (a painful, recurring skin condition) has improved, along with my mood, anxiety and gut health.

Before the Dirty Diet, I tended to avoid bread as it bloated me and made me lethargic. I had minimal dairy and what I did have was low fat, believing this could exacerbate my rosacea and congestion. I am now more regular, and am enjoying sourdough bread and loving Greek yogurt. I've increased the amount of fruit and veg I eat, and have added bread and cheese and rice in measured amounts without feeling they're bad for me.

This isn't just a diet: it's a way of life. I've been looking at my old diet books, and there's so much 'don't eat this, cut out this, detox the first week . . .' Ugh – that's why I never did them! The Dirty Diet was much more enjoyable. There are suggestions about things like cutting out sweeteners, but no hard-and-fast rules, as it's always about being sustainable.

Health changes: I achieved all my goals: my gut health has improved, I've had no rosacea flare-ups or sinus issues. I also didn't think monitoring my mood and anxiety was that relevant to me – until I saw my replies after four weeks, and the change has really surprised me!

I am so very happy with both my weight loss and flatter stomach.

Top tips: Try the recipes – I am addicted to the Waldorf Muffins and love creating my own versions. And my husband loves the Dirty Rice, Beef, Mushroom and Cashew Stir Fry, and Sticky Ginger Chicken.

T is for Training yourself in healthy habits

Quick fixes are all very well, but they rarely last. The Dirty Diet is about making changes that will last a lifetime. And part of achieving that is to understand which habits are damaging, and training yourself to replace them with better ones.

Your best personal trainer? Yourself!

No one else understands you as well as you do. It's not just your microbiome that's the result of the different things that have happened during your life. Your attitude to diet, your fitness habits, your cravings and your emotional triggers are all linked to past experiences. So it makes sense that you're the best person to make change happen.

The Dirty Diet tackles your cravings, rather than ignoring them

Losing weight and/or making dietary changes can be hard, for emotional as well as physical reasons. In the Dirty Diet, we encourage you to analyse those reasons and find ways to combat them. So in Part 2, you will draw up a Blueprint and look at the mental and physical struggles you have with your weight, health and fitness, and examine different strategies to deal with them. There is a science to creating more positive habits – you'll find more information about this in Part 2, from p. 96.

> Filling out the Blueprint definitely helped because it showed clearly what my personal cravings and triggers were, so I could see what I needed to do to rectify them.
>
> Summer, 20, student, Lancashire, UK

Learning from the world's healthiest people

For me, quality of life and health are as important as the number of years I live. If *your* aim is to maximise your health span as well as your lifespan – to stay as fit, active and pain-free for as long as possible – then you can learn from the people who manage both. So the broader principles of the Dirty Diet are based around studies of people who do live long, healthy lives.

Obesity has become a major crisis in the last few decades – yet in areas where traditional diets are still common – from parts of the Mediterranean to Japan and Costa Rica – people live longer lives and healthier lives. The research community has been focused on the 'Med diet' for decades, but now they're also looking at other pockets of good health around the world. Dan Buettner in particular has made a study of what he calls the Blue Zones® – five regions where he identified:

- More people living to 100 or even greater ages.
- People who were less affected by physical ill health and chronic conditions like type 2 diabetes, heart disease and stroke.
- People who didn't develop dementia, or only did so much later than the norm in most countries.

These are areas with very different diets and environments, yet there are common themes and habits that are applicable whether you live in the city, in the country or by the sea. It's not only about *what* these healthy populations eat – it's also how they live.

- Their diet contains loads of plants: they love their greens (and yellows and reds and purples). The deeper the colour the better – whether it's dark green spinach, blue-black berries, or glossy red peppers.
- They use good fats in cooking and on the plate – olive oil, oil-rich nuts, and fresh fish that's rich in Omega-3 fatty acids.
- They consume less protein from meat, more from plant and dairy sources like beans, soya, tofu, cheese and yogurt.
- They enjoy small quantities of nutrient-rich treats (including red wine and chocolate).
- They live balanced lives where they stay physically active during the day.

- They also maintain close relationships with family or through shared interests or faith.

That final point can also help you make successful changes in habits. Aim to spend time with people who want the same things – and that can include being part of an online community like our Facebook group where we're all aiming to adopt a healthier lifestyle.

These dietary habits are *very* similar to those that we know help the gut bacteria thrive. So a healthy microbiome could be a key factor in *why* these populations stay fitter for longer.

THE DIRTY DIET TAKEOUT:
T is for Training yourself in healthy habits

- Breaking habits and training yourself in better ones will make this diet last.
- The key elements in healthy eating – eating lots of fresh produce, less animal proteins and fats, more healthy fats and treats in smaller amounts – are common worldwide but can be adapted to suit many different diets.
- Using the tips to help you form healthier habits can increase your chances of making long-term positive changes.

THE DIRTY DIET IN ACTION
'It's all about sustainable habits'

Quinton, 27, IT technician, Durban, South Africa

After 28 days: lost 10lbs (4.5kg), 24.9 BMI (down from 26.2), more diverse diet, higher self-esteem

Quinton says: the Dirty Diet has really worked for me – I feel so much healthier, it's working far better than any other diet I've ever tried. I have been able to get myself onto a much healthier path in how I eat, my wife is happier because I am eating better, and the Dirty Diet has really been an interesting new way of life which will honestly be a pleasure for me to sustain! I still want to lose a bit more weight, but I am extremely happy with my current progress and I will definitely continue with the Dirty Diet as this plan really works for me.

Before the Dirty Diet, I had tried a local diet called Verslank met brood (Afrikaans for 'slimming with bread') which I used prior to getting married, to get down to around 82kg, but that was an intensely restrictive diet which was not at all sustainable in the long term. From there, I sort of gave up on dieting and fully embraced 'married life' – which ended up with me weighing over 100kg.

I have started eating more fruits, vegetables and salads. Prior to the Dirty Diet, I almost never ate salad (unless it was in a hamburger), but now I actually eat a side salad with most meals.

Health changes: Since starting, I have lost not only weight, but measurements as well, and I am really feeling healthier. The only difficulty I had was trying to ensure I ate a minimum of five portions of fruit and veg per day. It took a bit of discipline, but I am a lot better at it now. I intend to carry on with the Dirty Diet in its entirety as it is a fun diet which has allowed me to change my eating habits, expand on my tastes, and I really feel better about myself.

Top Tips: Drink as much water as possible, and if you don't like plain water, put freshly sliced lemon in the bottle – it is incredibly refreshing, and the change in taste helps. If you're busy at work and don't have time to cook fresh food every day, then cook at the weekend and freeze. I did that with some of my meals, and I found that it helped on those days when I got home late from work and wasn't in the mood to cook. It works really well with dishes like lasagne, curries, pies and quiches.

Y is for You

Our final principle is the most important for long-term success: this diet revolves around YOU, your weight loss and health priorities.

We're all individuals, yet too many plans fail to take that into account. Here are some of the reasons why most diets and lifestyle changes don't work or don't last – and why the Dirty Diet's personalisation helps make it different:

Our size, weight and calorie needs are not the same

Many diets are based on 'average' men and women – yet there's not really any such thing. In the Dirty Diet, you calculate your personalised energy needs, and pick meals and eating patterns to suit those. The meal plans do have suggested calorie guidelines but you can tweak to match your needs.

Your genes, gut microbiome and dieting history affect your biology

We encourage steps that improve gut health *and* observation of what approaches to healthy eating have worked for you in the past, to build a unique plan.

Your likes, dislikes and any allergies or intolerances aren't factored into strict plans

The foods I love could be your worst nightmare. The Dirty Diet offers suggested meals, but there's flexibility to fit your own tastes and lifestyle.

Everyone has different levels of motivation

How do you personally balance results vs effort? Some of us want immediate weight loss and want to go all out to achieve it, others prefer a steadier approach. The Dirty Diet allows for that by letting you choose your pace and your goals.

The reason intermittent fasting has worked for so many people in so many different countries and cultures is its flexibility. With the Dirty Diet, we're taking personalisation further, to draw up a Blueprint. The more you know about what makes you tick, the more likely you are to make long-term change.

I personalised a lot because my calorie needs were lower at first: partly because I had stopped exercising due to my weight, and partly because I'm 53. But I've now tweaked it a bit as I am exercising again now – mainly as I feel better in my swimwear. Living in Dubai, I am now back doing Aqua spinning under the stars.

Jane

THE DIRTY DIET TAKEOUT:
Y is for You

- Our calorie needs and our goals vary from person to person – understanding those helps you personalise the plan.
- The more you tailor the diet to your likes and dislikes, the more sustainable it will be.

THE DIRTY DIET IN ACTION
'The emphasis is on you as an individual'

Bridget, 62, tutor and writer from Brighton, UK

After 28 days: lost 15.5lbs (7kg), 40 BMI (down from 42.9), IBS improved and eating better than before.

Bridget says: After failing at every diet – and even seeing a hospital dietitian, this is the best diet I've ever been on. I like the fact that it's not faddy. I like the expertise behind it. I love the fact that it doesn't preach.

I'm on a diet and I'm eating better than I did before, and by better I don't just mean more balanced, etc. I'm eating tasty food. If I am being careful about the number of calories I consume, I want the ones I eat to taste nice, to add to the pleasure of eating. I am not going to live in purgatory for the rest of my life – a refusal to do so is probably why I failed at so many diets in the past. I'm no martyr. It really has made me enjoy food more. I don't feel eating is something I should feel guilty about because it's under control.

This is the first diet that made sense to me, because there is so much emphasis on me as an individual. I don't have to fit into a one-size-fits-all way of living. For example, one of my problems is that over the years I've learnt to ignore the feeling-full trigger that encourages you to stop eating. If there's a buffet in front of me I can just plough on, and on. So, making me eat breakfast when I don't want it or need it is forcing me to eat an extra meal, because I will go on to eat/want the same amount at lunch and dinner regardless. I loved the fact that I was given permission to skip breakfast by the Dirty Diet, recognising that that's the eating pattern I prefer.

The diet also makes sense because of the focus on the digestive system. I like the idea that it needs a break in order to work properly and that to keep consuming during your waking hours isn't giving it sufficient time to do its job. But perhaps the most sensible aspect of this diet is the emphasis on eating well.

Health changes: There has been an improvement in my IBS.

Top tips: I love bread. When bad things happen my hand automatically reaches for the bread bin. I have cut down on just having a slice whenever I was in the kitchen (and I work from home!) by buying a pre-sliced sourdough loaf and freezing it. I then toast from frozen a few slices as part of a planned meal.

Dirty great principles!

Those are our principles – understanding why we're asking you to do different things will help you make the right choices. If you have time to read more about fasting, the microbiome, digestion and traditional diets, there are details of useful books in the resources section in Part 4.

But now it's time to turn the principles and research into something that will work for you, for life. Turn the page to start work on *your* Dirty Diet Blueprint.

Part 2:
Your Dirty Diet Blueprint

Create a Blueprint to help you work out what you want – and how to get it!

It's time to get personal: use this section to fit the Dirty Diet to your lifestyle, your likes and dislikes, and your goals. You can make changes for life!

Use the questionnaires to discover:

- Your current energy needs and health issues;
- Your goals and motivations;
- Strategies for success and ways to build good habits.

This will add up to your Dirty Diet Blueprint – which will help you achieve life-changing results that last.

3 Steps to Creating your Dirty Diet Blueprint

Personalising the Dirty Diet is easy and enjoyable. Work through this chapter – you can also download a printable copy from the Dirty Diet website.

There are three stages to the questionnaire:

1. You today: your weight, measurements, calorie needs, habits and symptoms.
2. You in the future: work out *why* you want this, and how to deal with the things that are stopping you.
3. Your action plan: your final goal and your stepping-stone goals for weight and health, your choice of plan.

The questionnaire doesn't have to be completed in one session, and if you're keen to get started on the Dirty Diet right away, take your measurements for 1, 2 and 3. Then go straight to p. ??? to choose either the **Steady** or **Speedy plan** and learn how to build in **Bliss Moments**! But the more questions you can answer, the better your plan will be.

Why do the Blueprint?

Some of our trial Dirty Dieters needed a little persuasion to fill in the Blueprint. Here are the key reasons why it's useful:

- It helps you to monitor your progress;
- It helps you to personalise your routines and needs – one size never fits all;
- It reinforces the idea that this approach is about much more than how you look – it can also transform how you feel and how well your body works.

It was a good way to focus on the journey ahead and the goals I had in mind, visualising what it would feel like once I got there.

Sarah

I filled it in and then didn't look at it again until after four weeks and was *very* surprised to see how much I had lost.

Sue, 62, retired, Sunshine Coast, Australia

It helps to become aware from the very beginning that our diet will affect all sorts of other factors as well as weight, such as mood and sleep pattern. I wouldn't have thought to monitor any of that if it hadn't been in the Blueprint. It's a good reminder that this is about overall health, not just how heavy we are or how slim we look.

Kim

First Stage:
You Today

**Fill in the answers on p. 362
or use the downloadable questionnaire.**

1. Calculate your daily and weekly calorie needs (TDEE) and your BMI

Food equals energy – and if we eat more than our body can use immediately, the body stores the excess, usually as fat. To lose weight, we need to cut back on our food intake so the body has to use the stored fat instead. But our energy needs are influenced by many factors.

- Men generally need more calories than women.
- We need fewer calories as we age.
- People who do manual work need more than those working in an office.
- The heavier you are, the more energy your body needs to carry your weight around!

It's a key reason the one-size-fits-all diets don't work. For example, women are often said to have an average calorie need of 2000 to stay a stable weight. But even though I'm active, I'm also small and in my forties, so my need is only around 1800 calories. If I ate 2000 calories every day, I'd gradually put on weight.

Your daily calorie needs are known as your **TDEE: Total Daily Energy Expenditure**. It's an estimate of how many calories you could eat every day without losing or gaining weight. The quickest way to do it is to go to the calculator at the 5-2dietbook.com/calculator (there are two different equations for TDEE so you may find small variations if you do it elsewhere).

You need your current **weight** and your **height**, in either metric or imperial measurements. You also need to include your activity levels, from sedentary to very active. If in doubt over which level to choose, go for the lower one.

The calculator will give your TDEE and also your BMI: Body Mass Index – a basic calculation of whether you are a healthy weight or not. You're aiming for a number between 18 and 25 (or between 18 and 23 for some ethnic groups) – lower, and you are underweight, higher and you're facing the increased health risks associated with being overweight or obese.

NB: BMI is a useful guideline but does have limitations: use it alongside the waist/height ratio calculation opposite.

To work out your weekly calorie needs, just **multiply your daily TDEE by 7**.

2. Take your measurements

Grab a tape measure and measure your chest/bust and hips – add your upper arm and mid-thigh if you like. Record those results on the form on page 362, along with your clothes size.

By the way, if you're shocked to see your measurements written down, I understand – I've been there. But remember this is the start of your journey to feeling better.

3. Work out your waist/height ratio

The bigger your waist, the more likely you are to have 'visceral' fat around vital organs, which is a risk factor for heart disease and type 2 diabetes. To measure your waist, take a tape measure and measure midway between the bottom of your ribcage and your hipbone. You're at greater risk if your waist measurement is more than half of your height – that means a figure of over 0.5. For example:

Waist (32 inches/81cm) ÷ Height (64 inches/162cm) = 0.5 (so, borderline)

4. Health concerns

This part of the questionnaire on p. 362–3 pinpoints health concerns, so you can monitor any improvements. Score each symptom 0–5: 0 for no symptoms, 5 for a constant problem that affects your quality of life severely. Jot down any notes on triggers or patterns.

If you wish, you can also fill in a food and symptoms diary before you start the Dirty Diet: see p. 354 for more information about apps to make this easy.

5. Your food habits and feelings about food

The emotional side of eating is neglected by those people who say losing weight is simply a matter of calories in vs calories used. But the reasons we eat are so much broader than just feeling hungry. Being aware of *your* reasons helps you challenge and improve your habits – the Training that makes the T in DIRTY. Think of yourself as an investigator into your own health and diet – what's your ultimate mission, and what's stopping you getting there? The more you can understand your own needs, the higher your chances of success!

For me, this is a delicate area. I don't have an eating disorder but, for decades, I did feel shame around my weight and the fact I seemed unable to do much about it long term. Even now I get cravings for certain foods, and overdo it on occasion. The difference is I notice it happening and take steps to prevent it. If it **still** happens, I don't feel as guilty about the occasional episode of eating too much toast because I've had a bad day.

As you fill in the questionnaire, **be gentle with yourself**. If you find it raises big issues for you, talk to your doctor or to the eating disorders charity Beat (www.b-eat.co.uk). Awareness of eating disorders is growing and there is help available. Remember, it's not a good idea to do any kind of eating plan without supervision or advice from specialists if you have a history of anorexia nervosa, bulimia nervosa or other diagnosed disorders.

Consider the following and add your answers to the questionnaire on p. 364:

- **Cravings**. Which are the foods you crave regularly? They might be the ones you just love the taste of, or, very often, the ones you want when you're feeling sad or lonely or tired. They might be general or very specific: ranging from bread, to a specific brand of chocolate, ice cream or alcohol.
- **Trigger foods**. These can overlap with cravings, but they're generally foods that you find you can't stop eating once you've started (in my case, it's buttered toast with peanut butter).

6. Dieting history

- What weight loss diets have you tried before, and how successful have they been?

- What did you find most difficult? Why do you think they didn't work long term?

Don't feel bad – try to see it as helping you learn so you succeed this time round.

Second Stage:
You in the Future

This stage involves imagining a time when you're happy with your weight and feel fantastic, physically and mentally and then making plans to achieve that.

The 10-minute motivation exercise

Find a quiet place where you won't be disturbed, plus a notebook and a pen. This exercise helps you focus on why you want to make a change.

- Take 10 deep breaths in and out.
- Think about how you'd like to be feeling, looking and acting after you've been successfully following this plan for a month, a year, even 10 years. Write down everything that comes into your mind.
- Keep asking yourself why it matters to you: what will the changes you want give you? If you want to weigh less, or have improved gut health, how will that improve your life? Add to your notes.
- Imagine you've already reached your goal. What does it feel like? Write this down too.

After you've written down all your ideas, re-read them and **pick up to three words or reasons that seem most important**. They might be health motivators, emotional motivators or life motivators: read on for more detail on each.

Health motivators

Our bodies function better at the right weight. Many people in my Facebook groups have reported improvements in chronic conditions, from type 2 diabetes to migraines, after losing weight. Your digestion will also improve if you follow the Dirty Diet. Of course, diet is not a substitute for medical treatment. But the kind of changes that might motivate you to get to your ideal weight include:

- Better mobility, less strain on your joints.
- Lower blood sugar, reduced blood pressure or reduced blood cholesterol levels.
- Weight loss that makes you eligible for restricted surgeries or treatments.
- Improvements in anxiety and depression symptoms.
- Knowing you've a reduced chance of developing obesity-related illness including some cancers, type 2 diabetes and heart disease.

Emotional motivators

Being overweight is tough emotionally – other people can be harsh or offer unwanted advice. And often we're our own worst critics. Imagine leaving all the guilt behind. Your list might include:

- Knowing you can take or leave food, and enjoying it when you do eat.
- Not worrying about other people judging you because you know you're at a healthy weight for you.
- Feeling body-confident as you pack to go on holiday or shop for a special occasion.
- Enjoying sports because your body responds as you want it to, with strength and stamina.

Life motivators

Think about how your life will be better on a practical level if you achieve your goals, for example:

- Playing more actively with the kids or grandkids.
- Looking your best on your wedding day.
- Applying for that high-profile job that you've lacked the confidence to apply for.
- Going on a walking holiday.
- Dancing confidently with friends.

Using your motivators

Look at the motivators that felt most powerful to you in the last exercise.

- Copy them onto a postcard or sticky note and pin it somewhere you'll see it every day: on the fridge door, perhaps, or the bathroom mirror.
- Or choose a picture, a photo or an object (e.g. a wedding invitation, a shell from your favourite beach) to represent

what you want to achieve. If you use a picture or a photo, save it to your phone or laptop.

- If you're feeling low or unmotivated, look at the picture or hold the object and take a few breaths, imagining how it'll **feel** to reach your goal and achieve the things you want. Focus on the emotions and sensations.
- Set yourself an automatic daily reminder by email – maybe with the number of days until a special event or a reminder of your goals – that you can read to start your day.

Strategies for cravings, trigger foods and training yourself in healthier habits

Whatever the needs and emotional issues around food that you identified in the First Stage, this section offers solutions.

WHAT OUR DIRTY DIETERS SAY

You might think that if you've had cravings for many years, they're with you for life. But trying out the strategies in this book *and* focusing on the foods that do you and your gut good achieves real results.

For me, the biggest and greatest difference is that I rarely get cravings now. If I give my gut the right foods, it is not sending out the 'craving signals' in the hope of getting what it needs. So not 'gorging on biscuits by mistake'. That feels really good.

Timo, 52, local government worker from Kent, UK

It gives me great pleasure to ignore all the biscuits/ sweets/cakes that we have at work. I used to graze every time I got a cup of coffee, but having avoided them for ages I now don't feel that need to stuff my face!

Judith, 51, nurse from Lincoln, UK

Craving and trigger busters

Whenever we make a change, there are moments, or whole days, where it's a challenge to avoid grabbing that snack, or overdoing it. **The time to plan for these moments is in advance**, not when you're in the middle of a craving. Read these strategies and pick one or more to use.

A: Stash it

If there's a high-energy craving or trigger food you struggle to resist, make sure it's not in view or easily available. The easiest way is not to buy it – and ask the people you live with not to buy it either, or at least not to eat it in front of you. Don't think of the food as 'bad' – just recognise that it makes sense to control your environment so it's not in easy reach. With some cravings or trigger foods, you're always going to struggle to resist temptation. So take the temptation away.

B: Schedule it

Enjoy a trigger food but in a limited way, e.g. instead of buying a packet of biscuits, only have one biscuit – a delicious, home-made cookie – once a week at your favourite café. Or go for breakfast with friends, where you can enjoy toast but won't be able to order more than a couple of slices.

C: Delay it

What could you do in the 10 minutes after a craving hits to delay the moment so the craving passes? Write a list of nice things to distract yourself with – read a magazine, dance to your favourite song, paint your nails, play a game on your phone.

D: Sub it

This works well for cravings. At a time when you're *not* feeling hungry, review the foods you crave and think of a healthier food, lower in calories, that offers a similar flavour or texture. Or one that naturally comes in limited portions. For example:

Ice cream subs	Home-made ice lolly made with fresh berries Banana ice: freeze peeled banana pieces and blend straight from the freezer in a processor with fresh fruit like raspberries or pineapple. Chilled strawberries, marinated in the fridge in a little fresh orange juice Iced yogurt (but check sugar content, it may be no healthier)
Chocolate subs	Fruit-and-nut-based raw bar with cocoa flavourings (these tend to be made in smaller portions and are more filling than conventional chocolate bars) Very, very dark chocolate (aim for 80–90% on the label) with very little sugar is delicious but hard to eat too much!
Crisp subs	Nuts and seeds (make up your own portions and eat slowly, rather than having an entire bag open, since these are nutritious but are high in calories) Popcorn (pop it yourself and add flavours like paprika, sea salt or cinnamon) Poppadoms (the cook-at-home variety, made in the microwave)

Cheese subs	Olives (in brine, not oil)
	Smaller (matchbox-sized) portion of strong cheese, cut in advance!

Find a buddy

Dieters who have support do better than those who don't, so a great overall strategy is to find people who can help you stay focused.

Are there family members or friends who have been supportive in the past? Not everyone is helpful, perhaps because talking about weight triggers their own emotional issues. Pick people who are on board with your health goals, and explain what you're trying to do. Ask before you start the diet if you can call or text for encouragement if you're faltering.

If you don't think there's anyone in your current network who can help, join the 5:2 or the Dirty Diet private groups on Facebook for brilliant, round-the-clock support from people experiencing the same thing. (And avoid talking to the saboteurs – a debate isn't helpful or positive.)

Habit forming for beginners

Habits are automatic behaviours – things we do without really thinking, because they've become part of our routine. Think about eating at certain times of the day, brushing your teeth, even the order that you put on or take off your clothes!

In the Dirty Diet we're aiming to replace damaging behaviours with better ones, so that it's automatic for you to choose a more nutritious option, or to respond to emotion or stress with a non-food reward.

The amount of time it takes to break a habit – and form a better one – is very personal, and depends on how central that old habit was to your life, or how rewarding the new habit might be. But one study suggested it takes around 66 days – so if you stay on the Dirty Diet for nine weeks, you should be sorted for life . . .

FRESH habit-forming

To help you, here are the elements that can help you adopt a new FRESH habit.

Let's use the example of including a daily probiotic in your life.

Focus on how adopting this new habit will improve your life: the motivators you identified earlier in this section will help with this!

Example: A portion of yogurt or kefir will help my digestion work better – so I'll feel better daily, my weight loss can be sustained, and I will be more confident.

Repetition: doing something frequently helps it become a pattern.

Example: I will always take my yogurt/kefir at the same time every day so it becomes second nature.

Ease/Enjoyment: make the habit as easy and enjoyable as you can so it's a pleasure to do.

Example: I will mix the kefir or yogurt with oats and some fruit the night before so it's ready for me. And I'll choose my favourite fruits – juicy blueberries – to make it extra enjoyable.

Signal or Reminder: create a physical signal you associate with the new behaviour, to make sure you're less likely to forget.

Example: I'll put it next to the milk so I remember to have it as I make my morning cup of tea. And I'll put a note for myself on the fridge door until I remember automatically.

Habit: what you want it to become!

You can use these same techniques for *any* habit, whether it's food-related or not.

Third Stage:
Your Action Plan

In this final stage, you're going to use your measurements and other insights to choose the right plan for you.

First, decide:

Your weight goal

What would you like to weigh/what size would you like to be at the end of this process?

Your goal could be:

- A weight that puts you just into 'healthy' BMI category (between 23 and 25, depending on your ethnic background).
- The weight at which you've felt happiest in the past.
- The size you were on your wedding day, for example, or at another memorable time when you felt that you were in great shape.

If you're doing the Dirty Diet for health reasons rather than to lose weight, then read the guidance on p. 313 about how to maintain.

Stepping-stone goals

If you have a lot of weight to lose, it's also helpful to set mini-goals. For example:

- Moving from the obese to the overweight category in the BMI chart.
- Reaching the 15-, 12- or 10-stone mark.
- Fitting into a favourite pair of jeans.

Your weight loss-pace goal

Our suggested goal is 1–2lbs/0.45–1kg per week, though if you haven't been on a weight loss diet before or for a while, the loss in the first couple of weeks may well be greater.

What affects the speed of weight loss?

Most weight loss comes from your body using fat stores to fill a deficit or 'calorie gap' between the energy your body needs and the energy you digest from food.

The TDEE is the figure estimating what you need to stay a stable weight. Studies suggest you need a deficit of around 3,500 calories to lose 1lb/0.45kg in weight, so you're aiming to create a deficit of at least that amount per week – though the 'smart harvest' strategies outlined in D is for Diverse Diet (see p. 28) will help boost that.

On the Dirty Diet, we're achieving the deficit or gap by:

- Eating significantly less than your calorie needs on your two or three Fast Days, plus
- Optionally, eating a little less than your calorie needs on your Plenty Days.

So the pace of weight loss will be influenced by:
- How many Fast Days you choose to do each week;
- How far you eat below TDEE, if you choose to, Plenty Days.

But it's not just about the maths. The plan you choose *has* to be sustainable. It's counterproductive to set really strict guidelines, then get bored and give up. That's why most diets fail. So be honest with yourself, and remember you can also vary your plan week by week.

There are two basic plans: Steady and Speedy

Steady Plan
- **5 Plenty Days at 1,800 calories**
- **2 Fast Days at 750 calories, 3 meals per day (or fewer if you wish)**

This approach is similar to the tried-and-tested 5:2 Diet. It's a gentle introduction to intermittent fasting, and is also useful for those who have a lot of weight to lose or who have a higher TDEE – for example, an active and young male, or someone looking to lose over 4 stone/25kg.

> I decided to try Steady as I felt 1,800/750 was a good split for me. I calculated my TDEE and found that actually I could have had around 200 calories more, but I was happy with my decision. I feel full enough with this limit (which is a nice feeling) and intend to stick to it, although it's nice to know I won't be doing massive harm if I do go over.
>
> Jenni

I used the Steady calorie guidance but with the Speedy balance of days (i.e. three Fast Days and four Plenty Days), and it really worked for me.

Quinton

A blend for me. Speedy on the first week then Steady (due to stuff going on in my life), then Speedy again.

Timo

Speedy Plan

- **4 Plenty Days at 1,500 calories**
- **3 Fast Days at 600 calories, 2–3 meals per day**

The Speedy Plan is a little more intense, with the aim of a faster weight loss pace. It might suit you if you want to see results quickly, before a special event, and also if you have a lower TDEE than average. You may also want to do this for one or two weeks out of the four, either as a kick-start, or once you're used to fasting. Again, you can tweak this to customise it.

I used Speedy from the very beginning as I am vertically challenged, which does make a big difference to my TDEE, and I didn't want to eat past that amount.

Helen B

I went Speedy. Initially it was because I wanted to give myself the best chance, and another deciding factor was having more to lose, but I have thought about it again recently and realised that I like 4:3 because if one of your Fast Days doesn't quite go according to plan, you can still do the other two properly!

Sarah

Optional customisation for both Steady and Speedy plans

Depending on your goals, you might like to tweak the basic plans in these ways:

Cut back on your calorie limits – but not by too much

- If your TDEE is lower than 1,800, you may want to tweak it a little – my TDEE is only around 1,850, so if I am trying to lose weight rather than maintain, I would cut my Plenty Days down to a 1,700-calorie limit, and my Fast Days to 600 for a slightly faster loss.
- I generally recommend going for no more than 100–300 calories less than your TDEE on Plenty Days, if you do want to kick-start the loss. It will still be a lot higher than most strict diets allow.
- This also allows for occasionally over-eating, like at weekends, for example, and also for any errors you might make in weighing your food and calculating energy consumption (also see p. 317 for an alternative, hassle-free way of monitoring your portion sizes).

Choose how many meals to have, and when to eat them

Limiting yourself to a maximum of three meals a day and cutting out snacks helps you to stay full without overdoing it. But you can also choose to include 'time-limited eating' or 16:8/14:10 in your Dirty Diet schedule. You may have read about this back on p. 45, but to recap, this means eating within a timed 'window' on Fast Days and/or Plenty Days. So you might only eat during a 8 or 10-hour period, by eating your first meal a little later and your last meal a little earlier. Or you might go from three meals a day to two (something I do at times).

Advantages of having fewer meals or eating 16:8

- You're maximising the 'fasting' period where your body can repair itself and call on fat reserves for energy.
- This may encourage faster weight loss.
- On a Fast Day, your two meals can be larger than three would be.
- It's a strategy for taking more control of snacking or late-night eating.

Disadvantages of having fewer meals or eating 16:8

- You may prefer three meals a day, or dislike changing your meal times.
- You may prefer not to skip breakfast (though for most of us, the dire health warnings about skipping it are generally lacking in evidence).

- You may have medication that must be taken with food several times a day – always take advice under these circumstances.

Both plans include Bliss Moments

In the introduction we mentioned the concept of Bliss Moments – building the foods you really enjoy into your personalised meal plan. So those could be:

- a glass of your favourite red wine with dinner;
- coffee and cake with friends;
- ice cream on the beach;
- the cheeseboard at your favourite restaurant.

Planning Bliss Moments into your life

It's all about awareness. Ideally the food shouldn't be a trigger or a craving food, so you can enjoy it without feeling the urge to overdo it. Here are some pointers on how to choose, and how not to overdo it!

- Look up the calories in your favourite foods or drinks – a glass of good red wine might be 175 calories, or that slice of cake might be 300 or many more. You can find most branded foods on nutracheck.co.uk or myfitnesspal.com, and you can also get an idea of averages for home- or restaurant-made dishes.
- Look at your calculations from p. 83 – realistically, how many of these can you fit into your week without undoing the calorie limit?

- Stay aware of portion sizes – three small pieces of different cheese on a cheeseboard will probably be more enjoyable than a huge slab of the same one!
- Now schedule the food into your week. And when the time comes, savour it and have the best quality you can afford. So, go and enjoy the cake sitting at the best table of the café, rather than on the run, where you hardly notice it.

And don't overlook the non-food moments that make you feel fab too: keep a list of those as rewards and treat yourself as often as you can. They don't have to be expensive. For example:

- a trip to the beach with your kids;
- a long, hot bath;
- reading the new book by your favourite writer;
- a sunset walk in the park.

Blueprint examples

Nadia, 50, is 14lbs/6kg overweight – she wants to lose at least a stone for her daughter's wedding in two months' time. Her TDEE is 1,950 calories, which gives her a total weekly calorie need of 13,650. Nadia knows that she wants to see results fast, so she's decided to go with the Speedy Plan for the first couple of weeks and see how she does. She has decided to up the Plenty Day limit a little, though, from 1,500 to 1,600. This will give her an overall calorie deficit of 5,450, so that gives an approximate weight loss of 1–2lb/0.45–0.9kg each week. Once she's on track, Nadia plans to mix between Steady and Speedy, to allow for her daughter's hen weekend and other events!

Daily calorie need	1,950kcal
Weekly calorie need	13,640
Current weight	11 stone
Current BMI	26.2
Dress/clothes size Chest/bust Hips Upper arm Mid-thigh	14 40 inches 39 inches 12 inches 22 inches
Waist circumference Waist/height ratio	31 inches 0.6

Target weight goal	lose 14lbs/under 10 stone
Target BMI	25
Target pace of loss	1–2lbs per week
Stepping-stone goals	lose half a stone/7lbs after 1 month
Speedy or Steady?	Speedy but Steady once losing to fit in with hen night!
Plenty Day calorie limit Fast Day calorie limit	1,600 600
Fast Days per week:	3 Fast Days per week at first
Meals per day Doing 16:8/10:14? Y/N	2 Yes
My motivators: Health Emotional Life	Lowered blood sugar and height/waist ratio Feeling fantastic in 'mother of the bride' photos Going on to start dancing again
Buddy: who will I call/text?	Daughter, Facebook group
Trigger foods/cravings and strategies	Bread and cakes: no bread in the house but not banned – toast still on menu for Sunday brunch with friends
My Bliss Moments: 1 food-related moment – when/calories 1+ non-food moments – when/what	Really good glass of red wine 2 x per week (175ml each time) Massage every fortnight when I've lost weight

Steve is 28, and the weight has really crept on since he started a new job with a longer commute and less physical activity. He's now 3 stone/19kg overweight and feels fat and unfit. He's measured the basics but will judge other measurements e.g. chest, hips, by how his clothes fit.

As he's young and tall, his TDEE is slightly higher than average at 2,500, giving him a weekly calorie need of 17,500. The Steady Plan with its two Fast Days and generous 1,800 allowance on Plenty Days will give him a good calorie gap of 7,000, so he is going to try that. Steve should lose at least 2lbs/0.9kg per week – and because he's never dieted before, he can probably expect even more. But because he loves his snacks, he's going to plan for some extra side dishes in case he finds giving up snacking a bit harder for the first week.

Daily calorie need	2,500
Weekly calorie need	17,500
Current weight	16 stone (3½ stone overweight)
Current BMI	30
Waist circumference Waist/height ratio	41 inches 0.6
Target weight goal	13 stone
Target BMI	25
Target pace of loss	2lbs per week
Stepping-stone goals	7lbs at a time – celebrate after each half stone lost!
Speedy or Steady?	Steady
Plenty Day calorie limit Fast Day calorie limit	1,800 750
Fast Days per week	2

Meals per day	3
Doing 16:8/10:14? Y/N	No
My motivators: Health Emotional Life	Less out of breath during football training Shorts less tight, less self-conscious when changing Booking a beach holiday to show off!
Buddy: who will I call/ text?	Girlfriend, best mate
Trigger foods/cravings and strategies	Takeaways: having healthier ready-made curry in fridge ready for after football
My Bliss Moments: 1 food-related moment – when/calories 1+ non-food moments – when/what	Night out with girlfriend on Saturday night at favourite Chinese restaurant – try other restaurants too, e.g. Japanese/sushi for microbiome! (900–1,100 calories) Live music night with best mate (allowing for 2 half-pints too!)

My Dirty Diet Blueprint

It's time to fill in your Dirty Diet Blueprint!

	Start date	After 4 weeks	After 8 weeks
Daily calorie need			
Weekly calorie need			
Weight			
BMI			
Dress/clothes size Chest/bust Hips Upper arm Mid-thigh			
Waist circumference Waist/height ratio			
Target weight goal			
Target BMI			

Target pace of loss			
Stepping-stone goals			
Speedy or Steady?			
Plenty Day calorie limit Fast Day calorie limit			
Fast Days per week			
Meals per day			
Doing 16:8/10:14? Y/N			
My motivators: Health Emotional Life			
Buddy: who will I call/ text?			
Trigger foods/cravings and strategies:			
My Bliss Moments: 1 food-related moment – when/calories 1+ non-food moments – when/what			

Monitoring your weight loss

Monitoring your weight is also important – though it doesn't mean being a slave to the scales. You know whether you'll be upset if your weight fluctuates if you weigh yourself. If the figures are a bit of a minefield for you, find a pair of jeans or dress that fits perfectly at your ideal weight and try it on as you progress with the Dirty Diet – they'll tell you for sure.

If you're comfortable with weighing yourself, once or twice a week is about right, at the same time of day.

Part 3:
The Dirty Diet Plans and Recipes

Eat well, feel fantastic

Armed with your Blueprint, you're now ready to begin to ditch the guilt, love your food and lose weight with the Dirty Diet.

In this section:

- Recap on the two plans, Steady and Speedy;
- Discover the range of fantastic foods you can eat with our sample meal planners;
- Find Dirty Diet recipes for breakfasts and brunches; soups and light meals; main dishes, sides and sweet things;
- Explore quick options and ideal portion sizes;
- Read up on ready-made meals and eating out.

If you haven't filled in your Blueprint yet, I would highly recommend that you go back to p. 110 to complete it, or at least record your current weight and calculate your TDEE before starting the plan.

The Plans and the Recipes

In this section you'll find:

- Sample meal plans for four weeks of the Steady and the Speedy plans: all the plans are **completely customisable**, or you can **design your own from scratch** using the Dirty Diet principles.
- **50+ recipes for your Fast Days and your Plenty days,** plus a comprehensive list of foods and portion sizes with calorie counts.

Making this suit you is important, so here you'll find guidelines on ready-prepared meals, eating out and other options (these are after the recipes, from p. 299).

Back on p 100, you chose between the Speedy and Steady plans. Both plans are based on these key guidelines:

- You'll eat at least seven types of vegetable and fruit per Plenty Day and at least five portions on a Fast Day.
- You'll also have a **daily serving of probiotic foods** – dairy or non-dairy yogurt or kefir and/or fermented vegetables.

You can buy these or make your own, or you can also consider buying probiotic supplements if you don't like or can't tolerate dairy or fermented vegetables.

- You can enjoy **'smart harvesting'** foods like **cheese, oats, nuts and seeds every day** (with non-dairy and nut alternatives).
- **Nothing is banned.** Tuck into varied foods including full-fat dairy, grains, bread, meat, fish, coffee, alcohol and 'treats'. But there's flexibility for allergy-sufferers, as well as for your own personal likes, dislikes and dietary restrictions (though part of the fun of the Dirty Diet is being more adventurous with new ingredients!).
- **Bliss Moments** – your favourite foods – are included. Whether you love wine, cake or pizza – you build those in every week, to help you love your food without the guilt.
- **The only 'rule' is to cut out snacking – and with our super-filling dishes,** you won't need to eat between meals. In addition, we strongly recommend you reduce and ideally cut out artificial sweeteners and watch out for emulsifiers, which do not help good gut health.

Remember, you can also switch plans – for example, do a Steady week followed by a Speedy week, if that suits your schedule. You can eat Fast Day meals in any pattern – as three smaller meals, or a brunch and a supper, as a lunch and dinner, or breakfast and then evening meal. There's much more information on fasting if you're new to it in the I is for Intermittent Fasting section (p. 67).

If you're a snacker by habit, try picking one of the smaller dishes/salads/soups from the recipe section or simply a piece of fruit to have on standby if you really have a craving for something mid-morning or afternoon. Snacking occasionally won't do too much harm, but it's a habit you want to break most of the time.

We ♥ fruit and veg:

how to eat more fresh food – and what to watch if you have IBS

**Eating a diverse diet is the first DIRTY principle
and the key is to increase the range of vegetables
and fruit you eat every day.**

You'll probably have heard recommendations to eat your 'five a day' – five portions of vegetables or fruit. In fact, most countries have now suggested we increase that to seven or even 10 a day for the many health benefits. The priority is to eat more vegetables – five to seven portions – with fruit as a smaller proportion – maybe two or three servings.

> It actually IS possible to have your five a day – and more! I'm learning to think far more about diversity and variety, and the whole family is benefiting from better meals. And I'm learning not to see cheese/nuts/a glass of wine as 'slipping', 'cheating' or 'bad', but simply enjoying the foods I love and incorporating them into that diversity.
>
> Lorna, 20, student from Yorkshire, UK

I think the biggest change in my diet has been in the diversity of what I am eating. I have far more vegetables and fruit now than I did before. I love the tip about trying to 'eat a rainbow' and choose different coloured foods.

Kim

But if even five portions seems daunting or you're worried about the cost, here are my tips:

Make a start

If you currently struggle to eat one or two portions of fruit or veg, start building up gradually. Remember, this is about training yourself in better habits, without it feeling like a punishment!

Write a list of vegetables and fruits you enjoy, or are willing to try. Now, look for ways to add at least one portion to each of your three meals a day. For example:

- Breakfast: add tomatoes, grilled mushrooms or baked beans (beans can count as one of your five) or one of the fruit portions to Overnight Power Oats (see recipe on p. 167).
- Lunch: include a big salad or some spinach or baby kale stirred into soup while heating, and a piece of fruit.
- Evening/main meal: add one or two portions of hot veg e.g. peas, sweetcorn, green beans, roasted peppers or other favourites.

Each week, increase your daily intake by one or two portions.

Make a rainbow

Diversity is the most important thing, so eating the rainbow – planning to have as many different colours of fruit and veg as possible each day – makes that easy. A plate of bright foods looks so appetising.

Make it seasonal

Seasonal produce tends to be cheaper, especially in markets or greengrocers, so this is a good way to keep costs down. Find out what's ripe right now at www.eattheseasons.co.uk.

Seasonal veg and fruit also tends to taste better, because it's higher in antioxidants and the phyto-chemicals that show in the wonderful colours.

Make it cheap and easy

Frozen, tinned, bottled and dried veg and fruit tend to be cheaper and, so long as they've been frozen or preserved quickly after picking, they retain a lot of their nutritional benefits and remain high in fibre. They also work out cheaper as they don't go off before you remember to use them, and preparation time tends to be quicker too.

Good frozen options include: spinach, roasted vegetables, peas, edamame beans, sweetcorn, mixed veg, berries (though strawberries do lose their texture so are best used in ices or smoothies rather than whole).

Good tinned, bottled and dried options include: pre-cooked beans, chickpeas, black beans and lentils, tinned tomatoes, roasted peppers, artichokes, olives, sun-dried tomatoes and peppers, dried mushrooms.

And don't forget probiotic vegetable preserves like kimchi and sauerkraut (see p. 294 for how to make them yourself).

Make it a priority

Moving towards eating your seven+ per day is probably the best single thing you can do in your diet. It benefits gut health, it's more filling, it's nutritious and it weans you off processed foods.

A note if you suffer from IBS

As we stated on p. 22, if you suffer from digestive issues, especially IBS, be aware that increasing the amount and variety of different fibre types in your diet can cause symptoms including increased wind/flatulence, bloating and/or diarrhoea. In addition, the beneficial bacteria in kefir can be challenging, so we advise starting with small portions.

I should add my own personal experience here. I've been a vegetarian all my adult life, and have also suffered from IBS on and off since my mid-teens (though the two didn't begin at the same time). So although I am a veggie, and therefore my diet is already fairly high in vegetables, I've increased the quantity and variety of fibre since starting the Dirty Diet. When I was first testing the recipes for this book, my fibre content went up even more, because I was trying out lots of different versions of the recipes, along with kefir and other types of fermented veg.

And, reader, I must be honest here: my gut didn't like it, at first.

I had an increase in gas and bloating, which could be uncomfortable – and my old 'friend' diarrhoea made an unwelcome return for a couple of days.

The problem wasn't the fibre, but the amount – one day I must have had 10+ portions and it was too much at once. So I cut back a little on some of the foods I know can be slightly more problematic for me (Brussels sprouts, I'm looking at you) and also ordered some probiotic supplements in the form of sachets that Helen recommended to me for my symptoms (you can find more information about supplements in the resources section on p. 318).

This approach made my IBS much more stable. While I always encourage diversity, I also recommend you listen to your body – as we know from p. 59, our gut microbiomes are as individual as we are, and though fibre is the key to good gut health, those bacteria do need time to adjust, and how long that takes will vary.

Helen says: As Kate has found, anyone with a sensitive gut will potentially experience some negative effects of increasing fibre and changing your eating pattern. This will settle with time, but the following tips can help for specific symptoms:

Bloating and wind: Limit your intake of beans and pulses, Brussels sprouts and cauliflower, which increase your gas production, as well as sugar-free mints and gum. Oats and linseeds (1 tablespoon a day) may help by providing some more gentle soluble fibre.

Diarrhoea: *Drink plenty of water to replace lost fluids, but make sure this is mostly caffeine free – limit tea, coffee or cola to three cups a day max. Avoid sugar-free sweets, mints, gum and drinks containing sorbitol, mannitol and xylitol. Make a note of how much fibre you can tolerate and increase this slowly as your gut adapts. Remember your food and symptoms by using a tracker such as the MySymptoms app or a pen-and-paper food diary.*

The meal plans

The meal plans that follow are satisfying, delicious and have plenty of options for all tastes. But remember, they're just the beginning – you can easily mix and match different Fast Day and Plenty Day recipes with your own favourite dishes, to suit your lifestyle and preferences.

As well as a calorie count, I also include information about how much protein each portion contains – Helen suggests you should always aim for at least 10g per main meal – and how many portions of vegetables or fruit a portion will give you.

You can download a spreadsheet from thedirty-diet.com to allow you to add in your choices and ensure you're hitting the right balance. You can also easily substitute ready-made meals including soups, sandwiches, salads and pre-packed dishes. Look at p. 299 for information on making the healthiest choices when it comes to ready meals.

You also want to factor in your **Bliss Moments,** which will be unique to you: the plans have suggested a count for these, but cross-check how many calories your own choice has. Look too at the guidance from p. 304 onwards for healthy choices when eating out, but remember even those choices can be higher in calories than your allowance. I'd always say that a life without enjoying good food and good company is not one most of us would choose, so you can be relaxed about this once or twice a week. But eating a takeaway or drinking a bottle of wine every night *won't* give you the weight loss you need. **It's your choice.** There are four weeks of Steady and Speedy meal plans, and each week celebrates the food of the four different seasons, but can be enjoyed any time of year! Focus on:

• The foods you enjoy;
• Variety;
• Getting prebiotics and probiotics into your diet (see the recipe section for advice on buying or making your own, and p. 320–23 for info on probiotic and prebiotic supplements);
• Considering a daily multivitamin and mineral supplement (see p. 318 for more on supplements).

Other things to know:

• The plans are focused on weight loss rather than maintenance (see the final section about staying Dirty for Life to see what to do next)
• Include probiotics and prebiotics (pp. 65 and 66) every day.
• We recommend you aim to cut out snacking altogether. But in the early days, the best option is to have an extra light meal, salad or probiotic portion on standby if required, as you get used to phasing out eating between meals. Snacking occasionally won't do too much harm, but it's a habit you want to break most of the time.

AUTUMN/WINTER

Steady – Plenty Days Meal Planner – 5 X 1800 per day

These are suggestions and, where alternatives are given, the calorie count may vary slightly: remember you can choose to eat your calories in 1, 2 or 3 meals! Or substitute the dishes here with ready-made soups/salads/stir fries/ready meals with similar calorie counts and veg content! In all the meals listed, the portions of veg/fruit are shown in brackets.

	BREAKFAST	LUNCH	DINNER	Probiotics/ protein incl. cheese, yogurt, beans
DAY 1	Mushroom rarebit & oven-baked tomatoes (2)	Leek and chickpea soup with blue cheese topping (2) & 1 medium seeded/ sourdough bread roll	Bacon, bean & spinach risotto (or porcini mushroom and leek risotto) (2)	25g blue cheese (or other flavourful cheese)
CALORIES (Total: 1775)	280	300	475	100
DAY 2	Heart-warmer porridge with banana, cinnamon & pecans (1)	Barley mustard veg pot (5) or warm puy lentil salad with emerald veg (2)	Speedy chicken (or paneer or tofu) tikka with 40g (uncooked weight) brown basmati rice (4)	80g full-fat Greek yogurt
CALORIES (Total: 1772)	306	354	462	100
DAY 3	Fuss-free eggs Florentine with spinach (1)	Pumpkin & lentil soup (2) with 1 medium seeded/ sourdough bread roll	Beef/tofu, mushroom and cashew nut stir fry with 40g (uncooked weight) brown basmati rice, (4-5)	1 extra egg or 100g baked beans
CALORIES (Total: 1734)	300	300	484	100

Grains: bread, oats, rice, barley & more	Nuts, seeds or good oils	Veg or salad on top of main meals	Fruit – berries, tree fruit	Bliss Moments	Veg/fruit portions
1 40g slice sourdough with breakfast	1 teaspoon each pumpkin & sunflower seeds, 2 brazil nuts	80g sugar snap peas, 1 red pepper (fresh or roasted)	100g blackberries, 1 small banana	Your Bliss Moments	10
100	100	70	150	200	
N/A as grains/carbs already included in all meals	2 brazil nuts, 3 walnuts	90g cooked spinach with ground spices, 80g baby sweetcorn	100g blueberries, 1 medium orange or blood orange	Your Bliss Moments	15 or 12
	100	100	150	200	
N/A as grains/carbs already included in all meals	9 almonds, 7 cashews	1 large mixed salad with lunch including dark leaves, onion, carrot, beetroot	1 medium grapefruit, 1 apple or pear	Your Bliss Moments	11 or 10
	100	100	150	200	

DAY 4	Mexican tomato scramble on toast (1)	Chilli-spiked veggie (vegan) Cottage Pie (4) OR Blue cheese, leek and potato souffle bake with 80g tomato salad dressed with balsamic vinegar (2)	Chicken pasta bake with ricotta and butternut squash (3) OR Barley mustard veg pot with sweet potato wedges (6)	50g tzatziki or 30g hummus + fermented vegetable pickle e.g. kimchi with lunch
CALORIES (Total: 1738)	308	300	480	100
DAY 5	Sweet potato bubble and squeak with blue cheese or horseradish (3) plus 1 poached egg	Chicken or veggie dirty rice with bacon or veggie sausage (2.5)	Smoked salmon and watercress spaghetti/ veggie sun-dried tomato or artichoke spaghetti with 60g mixed salad dressed with 1 teaspoon olive oil & 1 teaspoon lemon juice/ wine vinegar (3)	150ml dairy or coconut kefir (with berries in smoothie if desired)
CALORIES (Total: 1759)	355	324	455	100

N/A as grains/carbs already included in all meals	2 brazil nuts, 3 walnuts	150g crudites with tzatziki or hummus, 30g salad leaves with dinner	100g raspberries, 1 medium apple	Your Bliss Moments	12 or 15
	100	100	150	200	
N/A as grains/carbs already included in all meals	9 almonds, 7 cashews	80g tenderstem broccoli, plus 1 grated carrot dressed in 1 teaspoon oil with lunch	100g mixed berries, 1 passion fruit	Your Bliss Moments	12
	100	100	150	175	

AUTUMN/WINTER		
Steady – Fast Days Meal Planner – 3 x 750 per day		
These are suggestions and, where alternatives are given, the calorie count may vary slightly: remember you can choose to eat your calories in 1, 2 or 3 meals! Or substitute the dishes here with ready-made soups/salads/stir fries/ ready meals with similar calorie counts and veg content! In all the meals listed, the portions of veg/fruit are shown in brackets.		
	Meal 1 300 calories	**Meal 2 300 calories**
DAY 1	Butter bean puttanesca with baked egg (2)	Chilli-spiked veggie (vegan) Cottage Pie (4) OR Blue cheese, leek and potato souffle bake with 80g tomato salad dressed with balsamic vinegar (2)
CALORIES (Total 730)	286	300
DAY 2	Overnight power oats with blackberry & apple or rhubarb and ginger (2)	Chicken dirty rice with bacon OR veggie dirty rice with veg sausage (2)
CALORIES (Total 759)	260	345

Light Meal 3/side dish/salad/soup	Green day 'free' probiotic	Veg/fruit portions
Leek and chickpea soup with blue cheese topping (2)	1 mini 'free' probiotic portion e.g. kefir shot from recipes section OR 2 heaped tablespoons fermented veg served with an oatcake biscuit or with a large pile of fresh spinach, rocket or other salad leaf	8 or 6
144		
Purple-sprouting broccoli with Romesco sauce (2) OR Pumpkin and lentil soup with herb butter/oil (2)	1 mini 'free' probiotic portion e.g. kefir shot from recipes section OR 2 heaped tablespoons fermented veg served with an oatcake biscuit or with a large pile of fresh spinach, rocket or other salad leaf	
154		

SPRING/SUMMER

Steady – Plenty Days Meal Planner – 4 x 1800 per day

These are suggestions and where alternatives are given, the calorie count may vary slightly: remember you can choose to eat your calories in 1, 2 or 3 meals! Or substitute the dishes here with ready-made soups/salads/stir fries/ready meals with similar calorie counts and veg content! In all the meals listed, the portions of veg/fruit are shown in brackets.

	BREAKFAST	LUNCH	DINNER	Probiotics/ protein incl. cheese, yogurt, beans
DAY 1	Greek yogurt fruit sundae with strawberries & nectarine, layered with choc-cherry granola (2)	Blue cheese and potato souffle bake with spring asparagus & 60g spinach and watercress salad dressed with balsamic vinegar (2)	Lamb meatballs with red slaw and 1 mini wholemeal pitta bread OR Mushroom and black bean koftas with slaw & 40g (uncooked weight) basmati rice (2–3)	150ml dairy or coconut kefir made into smoothie with fruit
CALORIES (Total 1794)	294	300	420	100
DAY 2	Fuss-free eggs with portobello mushrooms with mustard sauce (1)	Sweet potato broad bean tortilla with 80g tomatoes dressed with sherry vinegar (2)	Filo tart with salmon (leave out if vegetarian), gruyère, watercress & roast tomatoes (1) with cauli & broccoli tabbouleh (3)	1 25g piece blue or strong cheese
CALORIES (Total 1738)	300	315	473	100
DAY 3	Waldorf muffin with 1 small apple & 20g extra blue cheese (1)	Punchy new potato salad with either egg, tuna or bacon (2)	Sticky ginger chicken or tofu with tumeric rice noodles(3)	Tablespoon fermented veg with 3 tablespoons cooked black beans or chick peas in the salad
CALORIES (Total 1730)	293	284	473	100

Grains: bread, oats, rice, barley & more	Nuts, seeds or good oils	Veg or salad on top of main meals	Fruit – berries, tree fruit, bright colours	Bliss moments – can be combined	Veg portions
1 medium sourdough roll and butter with lunch	2 brazil nuts, 3 walnuts	80g Tenderstem broccoli & 80g baby sweetcorn, steamed	80g strawberries & 1 medium banana	Your Bliss Moments	12 or 13
150	100	100	130	200	
1 bread roll or 40g (uncooked weight) freekeh/other grain with lunch	9 almonds, 7 cashews	1/2 small avocado, 60g rocket or baby spinach	1/2 medium mango with 2 passion fruit	Your Bliss Moments	11
	100	150	100	200	
N/A as grains/carbs already included in all meals	4 small pecans, 10 pistachios	80g steamed asparagus, 1 roasted pepper	2 portions	Your Bliss Moments	10
	100	80	150	250	

DAY 4	Butterbean Puttanesca with baked egg (2)	Mushroom and tofu stroganoff (3)	Revved-up avocado and chicken caesar salad with parmesan kefir dressing (3)	80g full-fat Greek yogurt
CALORIES (Total 1766)	286	303	457	100
DAY 5	Avocado toast with feta, lime & chilli (1.5)	Sesame prawn/tofu noodle salad with crunch veg (3)	Middle-eastern veggie flatbread pizza (4) OR Hot devil flatbread pizza (2.5) PLUS Kale, pea and pesto salad (1.5)	50ml live Tzatziki or 30ml hummus with fermented veg
CALORIES (Total 1769)	322	342	455	100

40g (uncooked weight) basmati rice with stroganoff	2 brazil nuts, 3 walnuts	160g steamed mixed veg e.g. cauliflower and broccoli or asparagus and green beans	80g fresh berries & 2 slices pineapple	Your Bliss Moments	12
140	100	80	100	200	
N/A as grains/carbs already included in all meals	1 teaspoon each pumpkin & sunflower seeds, 2 brazil nus	2 grilled field mushrooms with 1 teaspoon olive oil, 3 sundried tomatoes or 1 roast pepper with breakfast	1 medium grapefruit, tablespoon pomegranate seeds, 10 cherries	Your Bliss Moments	14 OR 12.5
	100	120	130	200	

SPRING/SUMMER

SPEEDY – Fast Days Meal Planner – 600 per day

These are suggestions and, where alternatives are given, the calorie count may vary slightly: remember you can choose to eat your calories in 1, 2 or 3 meals! Or substitute the dishes here with ready-made soups/salads/stir fries/ready meals with similar calorie counts and veg content! In all the meals listed, the portions of veg/fruit are shown in brackets.

	Meal 1 300 calories	Meal 2 300 calories or 2 x Lighter meals
DAY 1	Butter bean puttanesca with baked egg (2)	Chilli-spiked veggie (vegan) cottage pie (4) OR 2 x soups/salads e.g. leek & chickpea soup AND egg pancake with blistered veg (3.5)
CALORIES (Total 586)	286	300
DAY 2	Overnight power oats with blackberry & apple or rhubarb and ginger (2)	Speedy chicken (or paneer or tofu) tikka (4) OR 2 x soups/salads e.g. Mexican smokey bean soup AND Broccoli & Cauli Tabbouleh (4)
CALORIES (Total 580)	260	320
DAY 3	Sweet potato bubble and squeak with blue cheese or horseradish (3)	Chicken or veggie dirty rice with bacon or veggie sausage (2.5) OR 2 x soups/salads e.g Thyme & sweet potato hummus & crudites AND Hot artichoke & pepper on sourdough (4)
CALORIES (Total 634)	289	345

Green day 'free' probiotic	Veg portions
1 mini 'free' probiotic portion e.g. kefir shot from recipes section OR 2 heaped tablespoons fermented veg served with an oatcake biscuit or with a large pile of fresh spinach, rocket or other salad leaf	6 or 5.5
1 mini 'free' probiotic portion e.g. kefir shot from recipes section OR 2 heaped tablespoons fermented veg served with an oatcake biscuit or with a large pile of fresh spinach, rocket or other salad leaf	6
1 mini 'free' probiotic portion e.g. kefir shot from recipes section OR 2 heaped tablespoons fermented veg served with an oatcake biscuit or with a large pile of fresh spinach, rocket or other salad leaf	5.5 or 7

SPRING/SUMMER

SPEEDY – Plenty Days Meal Planner – 4 x 1500 per day

These are suggestions and, where alternatives are given, the calorie count may vary slightly: remember you can choose to eat your calories in 1, 2 or 3 meals! Or substitute the dishes here with ready-made soups/salads/stir fries/ready meals with similar calorie counts and veg content! In all the meals listed, the portions of veg/fruit are shown in brackets.

	BREAKFAST/ MEAL 1: 300 CALORIES	LUNCH/ MEAL 2: 300 CALORIES	DINNER/ MEAL 3: 450 CALORIES	Probiotics/ non-meat protein incl. cheese, yogurt, beans, tofu, fish 100 CALORIES
DAY 1	Greek yogurt fruit sundae with strawberries & nectarine, layered with choc-cherry granola (2)	Blue cheese and potato souffle bake with spring asparagus & 60g spinach and watercress salad dressed with balsamic vinegar (2)	Sticky ginger chicken or tofu with tumeric rice noodles(3)	Tablespoon fermented veg with 3 tablespoons cooked black beans or chickpeas in the salad
CALORIES (Total 1492	294	300	473	100
DAY 2	Fuss-free eggs with portobello mushrooms with mustard sauce (1)	Lamb meatballs with red slaw OR mushroom and black bean koftas with slaw (add rice or pitta bread from grains if liked)	Middle-eastern veggie flatbread pizza (4) OR Hot devil flatbread pizza (2.5) PLUS Kale, pea and pesto salad (1.5)	50ml live tzatziki or 30ml hummus with fermented veg
CALORIES (Total 1499)	300	354	455	100

Choice of grains or Bliss Moments: 50g sourdough bread with 1 teaspoon butter/40g weight oats, rice, barley & more OR Bliss Moments: 150 CALORIES	Nuts, seeds or good oils as toppings or with dishes: 50 CALORIES	1–2 portions veg or salad on top of main meals: 75 CALORIES	1–2 portions Fruit – berries, tree fruit, bright colours: 75 CALORIES	Veg portions
Your Bliss Moment	2 small brazil nuts	160g steamed mixed veg e.g. cauliflower and broccoli or asparagus and green beans	½ small mango or 3 slices pineapple	9
150	40	75	60	
Rice with lunch or your Bliss Moment	8 almonds	1 roast pepper or 80g tomatoes	1 small banana	10.5 or 10
125	50	35	80	

DAY 3	Waldorf muffin with 1 small apple & 20g extra blue cheese (1)	Sweet potato broad bean tortilla with 80g tomatoes dressed with sherry vinegar (2)	Revved-up avocado and chicken caesar salad with parmesan kefir dressing (3)	1 25g piece blue or strong cheese
CALORIES (Total 1471)	294	315	457	100
DAY 4	Avocado toast with feta, lime & chilli (1.5)	Sesame prawn/ tofu noodle salad with crunch veg (3)	Filo tart with salmon (leave out for veggies), gruyère, watercress & roast tomatoes (1) with cauli & broccoli tabbouleh (3)	150ml dairy or coconut kefir made into smoothie with fruit or 80ml Greek yogurt
CALORIES (Total 1474)	322	342	475	100

Small Bliss Moment or oatcake with cheese	1 walnut, 2 small brazils	2 grilled field mushrooms with 1 teaspoon olive oil, 3 sundried tomatoes or 1 roast pepper with breakfast	1 kiwi, 30g raspberries	9
60	50	120	75	
Small Bliss Moment	1½ teaspoons mixed seeds	60g rocket or baby spinach with 80g sliced tomatoes, dressed with balsamic	80g strawberries with 1 passionfruit	
60	50	50	75	

AUTUMN/WINTER

SPEEDY – Plenty Days Meal Planner – 4 x 1500 per day

These are suggestions and where alternatives are given, the calorie count may vary slightly: remember you can choose to eat your calories in 1, 2 or 3 meals! Or substitute the dishes here with ready-made soups/salads/stir fries/ready meals with similar calorie counts and veg content! In all the meals listed, the portions of veg/fruit are shown in brackets.

	BREAKFAST/ MEAL 1: 300 CALORIES	LUNCH/ MEAL 2: 300 CALORIES	DINNER/ MEAL 3: 450 CALORIES	Probiotics/ non-meat protein incl. cheese, yogurt, beans, tofu, fish 100 CALORIES
DAY 1	Mushroom rarebit & oven-baked tomatoes (2)	Leek and chickpea soup with blue cheese topping (2) & 1 small seeded/ sourdough bread roll	Bacon, bean & spinach risotto (or porcini mushroom and leek risotto) – (2)	80ml full-fat Greek yogurt or 1 25g piece blue or strong cheese
CALORIES (Total 1460)	280	250	475	100
DAY 2	Heart-warmer porridge with banana, cinnamon & pecans (1)	Vegetable barley pot (5) or warm puy lentil salad with emerald veg (2)	Beef/tofu, mushroom and cashew nut stir fry with 40g (uncooked weight) brown basmati rice (4–5)	150ml dairy or coconut kefir, 1 teaspoon chia or oats, blended into smoothie with berries from fruit portion
CALORIES (Total 1515)	306	355	484	100

Choice of grains or Bliss Moments: 40g bread/40g weight oats, rice, barley & more OR Bliss Moments: 150 CALORIES	Nuts, seeds or good oils as toppings or with dishes: 50 CALORIES	1–2 portions veg or salad on top of main meals: 75 CALORIES	1–2 portions fruit – berries, tree fruit, bright colours: 75 CALORIES	Veg portions
Bliss Moment of your choice or toast with breakfast	1 walnut, 2 small brazils	1 large mixed salad with lunch including dark leaves, onion, grated carrot, beetroot, pepper, dressed with 1 teaspoon olive oil and a little lemon juice	1 small banana	9
100	50	125	80	
Bliss Moment of your choice or extra porridge	8 almonds	140g mixed steamed veg e.g. broccoli/cauli or fine beans and baby corn	100g mixed berries	11 or 10
100	50	75	45	

DAY 3	Your CHOICE e.g. Fuss-free eggs Florentine with spinach (1)	Chilli-spiked veggie (vegan) cottage pie (4) OR Blue cheese, leek and potato souffle bake with 80g tomato salad dressed with balsamic vinegar (2)	Speedy chicken (or paneer or tofu) tikka with 40g (uncooked weight) brown basmati rice (4)	50ml live yogurt tzatziki or 30g hummus with fermented veg pickle
CALORIES (Total 1487)	300	300	462	100
DAY 4	Mexican tomato scramble on toast (1)	Chicken or veggie dirty rice with bacon or veggie sausage (2.5)	Smoked salmon and watercress spaghetti/ veggie sun-dried tomato or artichoke spaghetti with 60g mixed salad dressed with 1 teaspoon olive oil & 1 teaspoon lemon juice/wine vinegar (3)	100g baked or cooked black beans with fermented veg with breakfast (1)
CALORIES (Total 1502)	308	324	455	100

Bliss Moment of your choice or slice of toast	1½ teaspoons mixed seeds	2 large field mushrooms grilled with ½ teaspoon olive oil & mixed herbs	1	11 or 9
125	50	75	75	
Bliss Moment of your choice	2 brazils	2 portions frozen veg with lunch e.g. 80g peas/beans, 80g spinach or sweetcorn	1 small apple or pear, 1 passion fruit	10
100	40	100	75	

A note on calorie-counting

Many people hate the idea of calorie-counting – but the good thing about the Dirty Diet is that this is only needed while you re-learn the foods your body needs, so long term you won't have to think about it at all. You might *think* you already know how much you're consuming, but the early days can be shocking – and enlightening!

For example, the serving size recommended on a cereal packet is probably much less than you usually pour. Weighing will help you discover where you might be adding 'hidden' calories.

I've always refused point-blank to calorie-count, but I felt I ought to give it a try because I was in the panel trying the Dirty Diet. Oh boy, was I in for a lesson! I really had no idea how much the little extras can add up, and now I do I am very mindful of everything I eat (e.g. eating 3–6 almonds, not the whole bag). A month counting calories was so worth it. I could have saved myself years of bad dieting if I had realised.

Sue

The good news is it's much simpler than before to count calories, by using free or low-cost apps. Try Nutracheck.co.uk if you're UK-based, or MyFitnessPal. I prefer the former as it is more accurate, but it does involve a small monthly fee – you can try it for a week for free, though. It's also a little mean when it comes to veg/fruit portions, so keep your own notes.

Calorie-counting on a Fast Day

Weigh your ingredients as you get used to Fast Day portion sizes. It doesn't take long – I keep small, cheap digital scales on the worktop and put a bowl or pan on top, using the 0 button and adding ingredients as I go.

Soon you'll be much more aware of what a portion size is, and which choices offer the most filling food for fewer calories. At that stage, you won't need to count any more.

Calorie-counting on a Plenty Day

The meal plans and recipes are already calorie-counted, so if you're following those all you need to do is make the food as instructed.

If you're adapting them, then you will need to keep an eye on the calories, but again, you'll soon be able to judge by eye what a healthy, filling portion size is.

Dirty Diet Recipes

Symbols

(symbol) – **vegetarian, or with vegetarian option**

(symbol) – **vegan, or with vegan option**

(symbol) – **gluten-free, or with gluten-free option**

(symbol) – **dairy-free, or with dairy-free option**

NB: When we refer to calories in the book, we actually mean kilocalories. In Australia and New Zealand, kilojoules are used on packaging – one kilocalorie is 4.1 kilojoules.

Most recipes either serve 1 person *or* can be made as a batch of up to 2–4 portions, to be kept in the fridge to be eaten during the week, or frozen. But, of course, it's easy to scale up to feed friends or family, once they've seen how tasty the Dirty Diet is . . .

Seasonings:

I haven't listed salt and pepper for seasoning in most recipes, but a sprinkling of freshly ground black pepper really peps up most savoury dishes. Although reducing the salt in our diet is a sensible goal, if you're reducing your intake of processed foods significantly, you can afford to add a little sea salt to home-made dishes unless you have high blood pressure. Alternative no-salt and low-calorie seasonings include fresh and dried herbs, lemon and lime juice and herb, wine or balsamic vinegars.

Breakfasts and brunches

These are all satisfying *and* delicious: some are very portable for when you're in a hurry, others perfect for a leisurely weekend brunch. To help get as much variety into your diet as possible, pick 3 different breakfasts, ideally including savoury *and* sweet options, and rotate them!

Portobello Mushroom Rarebit with Oven-Baked Tomatoes

280 calories, 16g protein, 2 portions of veg

This is a delicious breakfast for both Fast Days and Plenty Days and the rarebit mix keeps in the fridge in a covered container for up to two days, so you can use it on anything else you fancy. It's great directly on toast or on top of a pre-cooked fillet of smoked fish, like haddock, finished off under the grill.

Serves 4 as a main
Preparation time: 5 minutes
Cooking time: 14–18 minutes

8 medium portobello mushrooms (around 50g each)
400g cherry or baby plum tomatoes
1 tsp oil

For the rarebit mix:
2 eggs
80g mature Lancashire cheese, finely crumbled or grated
2 tbsp stout or semi-skimmed milk
2 tsp English mustard
1 small red onion, finely chopped

To serve:
4 x 50g slices sourdough or gluten-free bread
50g rocket or dark leaves

1. Preheat the oven to 200°C/180°C fan/400°F/Gas mark 6. Wipe the mushrooms and remove very woody stalks. Halve the cherry tomatoes and place cut side up in an ovenproof dish, then put the mushrooms on top, gill-side up. Brush with a little oil and bake till the mushrooms have just softened (the biggest mushrooms may take a little longer), around 8–10 minutes.
2. Meanwhile, prepare the rarebit mix. Beat the eggs with a fork in a small bowl. Add the cheese followed by the stout/milk, mustard and onion and mix well. Season well.
3. Spoon the egg mixture on top of the mushrooms (if they've released a lot of liquid, pour this off the baking tray first). Place back in the oven for 6–8 minutes, until the cheese mixture puffs up and browns, but don't let it burn.
4. Toast the bread and serve the mushrooms on top, garnished with the salad leaves.

VARIATION: You could use pesto instead of mustard (1 tsp of shop-bought pesto is around 23 calories, depending on brand).

PLENTY DAY SUGGESTIONS: Serve with extra toast, or add 25g of cooked ham to the rarebit mix.

Butter Bean Puttanesca with a Baked Egg

286 calories, 18g protein, 2 portions of veg

The flavours in this dish really work – the soft, bland butter beans, the strong Italian additions, and the richness of the egg. You can cut the time right down by using tinned beans if you like, and if you worry about onion and garlic at breakfast, leave them out and use a few more capers and an extra chilli – if you can take the heat.

Serves 4

Preparation time: 10 minutes (plus overnight soaking)

Cooking time: 35–45 minutes for the beans, 10–12 minutes for the eggs

200g butter beans, dried, uncooked

5g butter or oil

1 red onion, diced

1 garlic clove, crushed or finely chopped

1 small chilli pepper, seeds removed, finely chopped

300g cherry tomatoes, roughly chopped

35g sun-dried tomatoes, roughly chopped

15 pitted black olives, in brine, drained, roughly chopped

2 tbsp tomato purée

15ml red wine vinegar or cider vinegar

15g capers

4 medium eggs

1. Put the butter beans in a bowl and cover with cold water. Soak overnight.
2. The next day, drain the soaked beans and rinse briefly. Gently heat the butter or oil in a saucepan and fry the onion, garlic and chilli for about 5 minutes until they've softened.
3. Now add the drained beans, and 600ml cold water. Boil for 10 minutes, then reduce the heat to a simmer for 15–25 minutes or until the skins and insides are just tender (this depends on the age of beans). Keep topping up the water, don't allow the pan to dry out.
4. Add the fresh tomatoes, sun-dried tomatoes and olives to the pan with the tomato purée, vinegar and capers. Top up the water if needed and cook for another 5 minutes. You can store the mix in the fridge, covered, till ready to use.
5. Preheat oven to 200°C/180°C fan/400°F/Gas mark 6. Layer a quarter of the mixture into 1 shallow ovenproof bowl/ tin per serving. Push down with the back of a spoon in the centre to make a dip, then break the egg into it. Bake for 10–12 minutes, till the egg white has solidified – you can also finish it off under the grill if the beans are already warm.

VARIATION: To make with tinned butter beans: Drain and add beans at the end of stage 2 and skip step 3, adding all the other flavouring ingredients from stage 4.

PLENTY DAY SUGGESTIONS: Serve with 2 slices of sourdough toast or add an extra egg. Sprinkle with Parmesan or Cheddar on top and grill till it bubbles.

Greek Yogurt Fruit Sundae with Choc-Cherry Granola

294 calories, 9.7g protein, 2 portions of fruit

This is such a delicious and adaptable breakfast option – the creaminess of the yogurt and the sweet-sharpness of fruit, with the crunch from the granola, make it one to savour. The granola is so easy to make but do watch serving sizes, as if you double up, you're also doubling up calories.

Serves 1

Preparation time: 3 minutes plus granola (see p. 156 for recipe)

100g full-fat Greek yogurt
1 portion organic fruits – choose from:
1 large peach or nectarine with 8 strawberries;
1 whole blood orange, chopped into segments, with 40g fresh raspberries;
100g cherries, weighed with stones in, with 100g slice honeydew melon;
or other fruit portion adding up to around 70 calories
1 portion (20g) Choc-Cherry Granola (see p. 156)

1. Slice or chop stone fruit (don't peel: the skin is good for you, but choose organic if you're going to eat it!) or wash and dry berries.

2. To serve, place the fruit in the bottom of a serving bowl or glass, add the yogurt and top with the granola. This can be done the night before for a very fast breakfast.

Choc-Cherry Granola

104 calories, 2.4g protein per serving

Makes 15 servings

1 tablespoon mild-flavoured olive oil

60ml honey or agave nectar

2 tsp unsweetened cocoa powder, e.g. Green and Black's

150g jumbo rolled oats

30g mixed seeds, e.g. pumpkin, sunflower, flax, sesame

45g almonds in their skins

75g dried cherries

1. Preheat the oven to 150°C/130 °C fan/300°F/Gas mark 2. In a bowl, mix the oil, honey or nectar and cocoa powder. Add the oats, seeds and almonds and mix so they are well coated with the syrup.
2. Line a baking sheet with non-stick baking parchment, spread the oats over it, and bake for 20 minutes. If the cherry pieces are larger, chop these, then add to the oats and bake for another 10 minutes. Let the granola cool down completely, then store in an airtight container. It will keep for a month or longer (though in my house it's generally eaten faster than that!)

VARIATIONS: The granola can be different every time: try with various dried fruits (e.g. chopped apricots, raisins – any mix with no added sugar). Leave out the cocoa and add vanilla, lemon or almond extract to the oil, or ground ginger or cinnamon as an extra flavouring. Other nuts like pistachios or cashews taste great too. With different ingredients, do keep an eye on the granola as it bakes to ensure it doesn't burn. Check oats are from a gluten-free factory if you are avoiding gluten.

Avocado Toast with Feta, Lime and Chilli

322 calories, 12.7g protein, 1.5 portions of veg

Super quick and easy – and just because avocados have become associated with some of the clean-eating extremes, it doesn't mean they're not delicious or good for you. I like them best with some crunchiness to offset the mellow, smooth flesh – toast is just perfect! Make sure it's ripe as unripe avocado isn't nice. Of course, this is an ideal breakfast for two.

Serves 1

Preparation time: 4 minutes

Per serving:

1 x 50g slice sourdough bread

½ ripe, medium avocado

Juice and zest of 1 lime

Salt and pepper

30g reduced-fat feta-style salad cheese (OR 10g Pumpkin seeds for vegan option)

1 fresh red chilli or a scattering of dried chilli flakes

30g pea shoots

1. Toast the bread.
2. Meanwhile, scoop the avocado flesh into a small bowl and mix with most of the lime juice (reserve a quarter-sized segment of lime for serving) and zest. Season well with salt and pepper.

3. Spread the avocado onto the toast, sprinkle over the feta or seeds and some of the pea shoots.
4. Serve with the lime segment and the rest of the pea shoots.

PLENTY DAY SUGGESTIONS: Use both the feta and pumpkin seeds and add a medium poached egg, plus a drizzle of 1 teaspoon olive or avocado oil, to bring up to 490 calories and 21.1g protein.

Waldorf Muffins with Blue Cheese, Apple and Walnuts

185 calories per muffin, 7.4g protein.

Blue cheese, apples and walnuts with a good dollop of oats: these are full of flavour and are great for taking with you for breakfast – in the meal plans we add 20g blue cheese and a small dessert apple, to give you a tasty, portable meal on the go, which is 293 calories and 11.4g protein. NB: These don't keep as well in a tin as sweet muffins, because the blue cheese can go mouldy out of the fridge! Instead, I recommend freezing: cool completely and freeze in a plastic box for up to one month. Defrost fully before serving.

Makes 12 muffins
Preparation time: 15 minutes
Cooking time: 20–25 minutes

50g wholewheat flour
150g self-raising white flour
1 tsp baking powder
½ tsp bicarbonate of soda
90g jumbo rolled oats
25g walnuts or pecans, lightly crushed
1 medium cooking apple, washed and cored, chopped into
100g blue cheese, crumbled
very small dice
2 medium eggs

150ml whole milk

100g full-fat Greek yogurt

For the topping:

10g walnuts, lightly crushed

10g oats

30g blue cheese

1. Preheat the oven to 180°C/160 °C fan/350°F/Gas mark 4. Line a 12-hole muffin tin with paper cases – you may want to use foil-lined ones, as the dough can stick to ordinary ones.

2. Sift the two flours together into a bowl with the baking powder and bicarbonate of soda. Add the oats, nuts, apple and blue cheese. Season (but go easy on salt as the cheese is quite salty). In another bowl, mix together the eggs, milk and yogurt. Add to the dry ingredients, mixing lightly with a spatula to combine – don't overmix or your muffins will be heavier.

3. Spoon mix into cases and then divide topping between the 12 muffins: I like to put the nuts and oats on first, with a piece of cheese on the top so it melts.

4. Bake for 25–30 minutes till well browned on top. Allow to cool on a rack. You can freeze these in a container and thaw overnight for breakfast.

PLENTY DAY SUGGESTIONS: 2 muffins plus the extra cheese and an apple as mentioned in the intro adds up to 478 calories. Or they're really good with soup!

Sweet Potato Bubble and Squeak Mash with Blue Cheese/Horseradish Sauce

289 calories, 9g protein, 3 portions of veg

Perfect for a Monday after a big Sunday roast, and although this is in the brunch section, it makes a very fine supper too. Lots of gut-friendly goodies here, and if you want a vegan version just leave out the blue cheese and use the horseradish sauce (but not horseradish cream, which does usually include dairy) or a little mustard. It works fine with normal spuds too.

Serves 2
Preparation time: 3 minutes
Cooking time: 10 minutes

1 medium baked or boiled sweet potato, around 240g raw
1 small red onion, diced
200g cooked greens: cabbage, kale, spring greens, Brussels sprouts, finely shredded
2 tsp butter or olive oil
25g blue cheese, crumbled, or 2 tsp horseradish sauce
100ml dairy or coconut kefir
2 sprigs fresh herbs, e.g. fresh thyme

1. Lightly mash the sweet potato: if it's been baked, include some of the soft skin for extra fibre.

2. Heat half of the butter or oil in a saucepan. Fry the onion and greens till they're just starting to brown, around 3 minutes. Add the potato and mix in the pan as they heat through and start to squeak!

3. Add the rest of the butter or oil to the pan and cook some more until the vegetables are completely warmed through and browning – you can choose to let it burn slightly in places if you like it. Turn in the pan so both sides of the mash are cooked, around 3–4 minutes on each side. Taste and season.

4. While the veg is cooking, whisk together the cheese or horseradish sauce, kefir and the leaves from the herbs (chop if they're larger).

5. To serve, divide the two portions onto two plates, pour the kefir sauce over the top and garnish with a few more herb sprigs.

PLENTY DAY SUGGESTIONS: This is outstanding with a poached egg or two on top, or a veggie or meat sausage.

Fuss-Free Eggs Florentine/ Benedict/Royale

300–325 calories, 14–18g protein

I first made this simple sauce a couple of years ago – it's easier and much healthier than the hollandaise sauce that usually goes with Eggs Benedict, Florentine and Royale. I still love hollandaise but it's too fiddly for me to make at home. This sauce, however, couldn't be quicker, and it works when you're on a Fast Day, or with extras on Plenty Days.

Serves 1
Preparation time: 5 minutes
Cooking time: 7 minutes

2 thin (25g each) slices of sourdough or wholegrain bread

1 medium egg

Splash of vinegar

For the sauce:

50ml half-fat crème fraîche

1 tsp Dijon mustard

Fresh herbs, e.g. chives, parsley or dill

Choose one of the following extras:

100g fresh or frozen spinach, ½ tsp melted butter, squeeze of lemon juice

OR 100g asparagus with ½ tsp melted butter

OR 25g smoked salmon, cut into pieces

OR 2 thin (15g each) slices of honey-roast ham

OR 2–3 portobello mushrooms (50g)

1. Make the sauce by heating the crème fraîche and mustard gently in a small saucepan for 2 minutes. Use scissors to snip the herbs directly into the saucepan, reserving a few leaves for garnish. Season to taste. If the sauce is too sharp for you, add a pinch of sugar.
2. Toast the bread lightly under the grill or in a toaster.
3. For the egg(s), bring a medium saucepan of water to the boil with a splash of vinegar. Break your egg into a cup. Create a whirlpool in the water with a fork or whisk and, with your other hand, slip the egg into the middle of the saucepan as gently as possible. Turn off the heat and set a timer for 3 minutes. After that time, check that the egg white has set before removing from the saucepan using a slotted spoon. Place gently onto a plate lined with kitchen paper to absorb the excess cooking water.
4. Extras:
   - For the spinach option, cook with a squeeze of lemon juice – squeeze all moisture out of spinach before serving topped with ½ tsp melted butter.
   - For the asparagus option, trim woody bases, then steam, boil or microwave for 2–8 minutes depending on whether the asparagus is fine or full-sized stalks. Serve with the melted butter.
   - For the mushrooms, remove the central stem if too woody, then dot with butter and grill or pan-fry on

both sides till cooked (around 2–3 minutes per side
depending on size).

5. Set the toast on a warm plate, lay the spinach, ham,
   salmon, asparagus or mushrooms on top, then add the
   egg(s) and finally the sauce. Season, garnish with the
   reserved herb leaves and serve immediately.

VARIATIONS: I like to top this with 10g blue cheese or add
a teaspoon of horseradish sauce, instead of or as well as the
mustard – it's really flexible. You can also make the sauce by
combining all the sauce ingredients and microwaving in a
small dish for 20–30 seconds, in 10-second bursts, stirring in
between.

PLENTY DAY SUGGESTIONS: Try adding an extra egg,
doubling up the veg or protein, and buttering your toast!

Overnight Power Oats with Fruit and Crunchy Nuts

260–300 calories, up to 9g protein, 2 portions of fruit

I am always raving about overnight oats (also called bircher muesli), as I much prefer the texture to hot porridge, and it's so quick to make. Make two or three portions in one go and keep, covered, in the fridge. You can leave out the nuts or seeds if you don't like them, but if you're not having dairy milk, I'd recommend adding the nuts to keep protein levels up. My favourite is the apple juice version.

Serves 1
Preparation time: 3 minutes

40g rolled or jumbo oats
125ml almond milk, semi-skimmed/skimmed milk or
unsweetened apple juice
Plus one fruit option and one nut option (see over)
50ml kefir (optional)

- Place the oats in a serving bowl (or plastic food container if you plan to take to work). Add the milk or juice and leave in the fridge overnight – or for a couple of hours at least.
- The next morning, or when it is ready to prepare, add fresh fruit and nuts, and top with kefir if using.

Fruit options: choose one

- 1 small banana and passion fruit seeds OR
- 15 raspberries (60g) and 10 strawberries (100g) plus a few drops of vanilla essence or 1 tbsp fresh orange juice OR
- 80g slice mango and 80g slice pineapple or melon, chopped OR
- 1 small apple, grated, and 75g blackberries OR
- 75g ginger rhubarb compote, see under variations below.

Nut options: choose one

- 1 tsp milled flaxseed and fruit mix, seeds or ground almonds OR
- 4 almonds OR 5 cashews OR 6 pistachios OR 2 walnut halves

VARIATIONS: To make 4 servings of ginger rhubarb compote: Use 300g rhubarb, 1 tsp ground ginger, 2 tbsp honey or agave nectar (or 40g sugar). Cook in a pan with enough water to cover till the rhubarb is soft. Keep covered in fridge for up to 1 week.

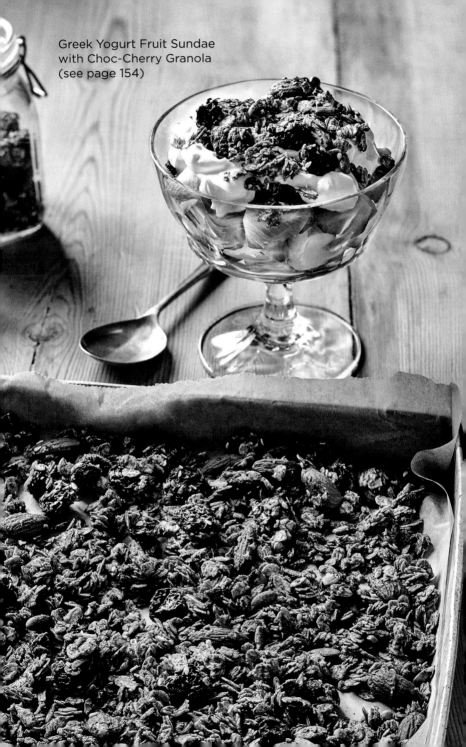

Greek Yogurt Fruit Sundae
with Choc-Cherry Granola
(see page 154)

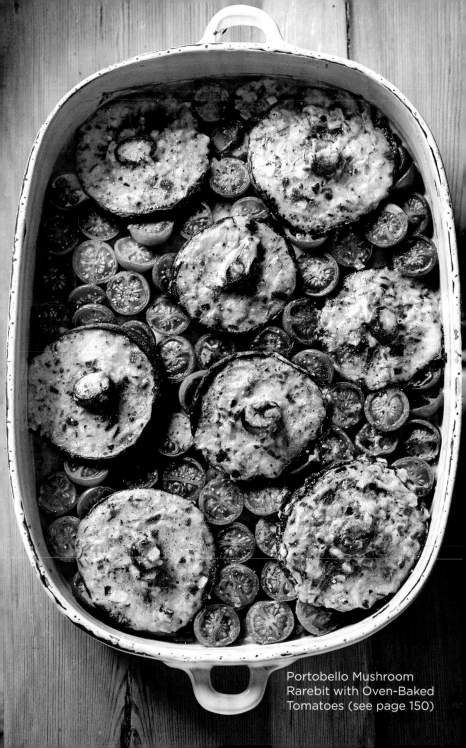

Portobello Mushroom
Rarebit with Oven-Baked
Tomatoes (see page 150)

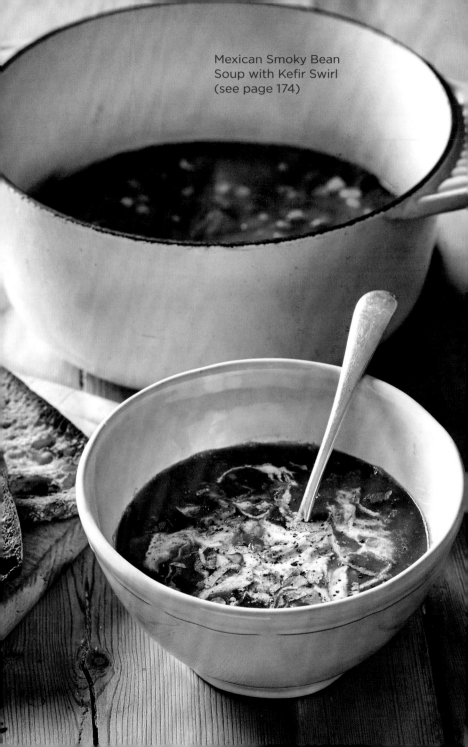

Mexican Smoky Bean
Soup with Kefir Swirl
(see page 174)

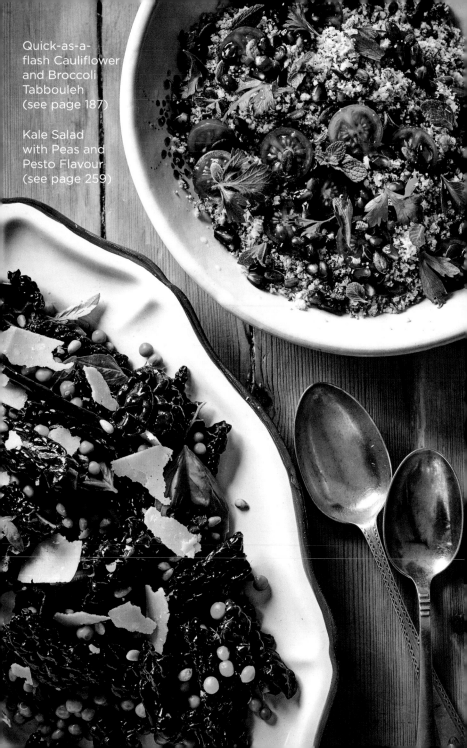

Quick-as-a-
flash Cauliflower
and Broccoli
Tabbouleh
(see page 187)

Kale Salad
with Peas and
Pesto Flavour
(see page 259)

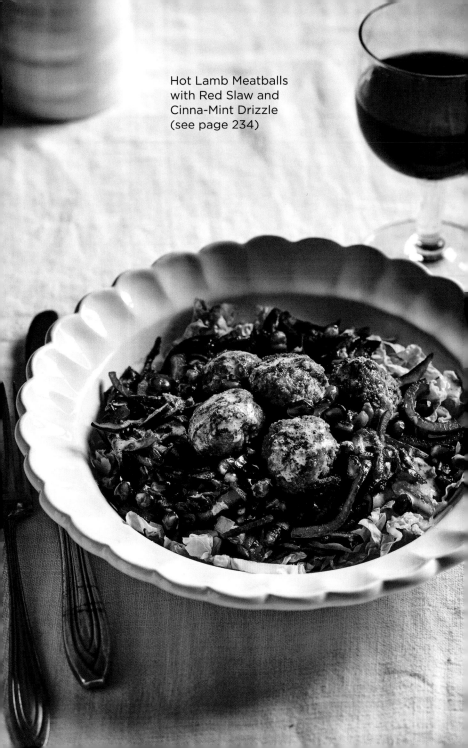

Hot Lamb Meatballs
with Red Slaw and
Cinna-Mint Drizzle
(see page 234)

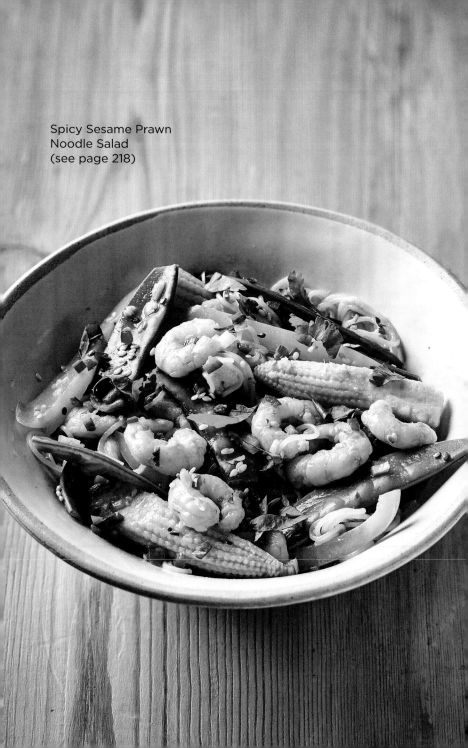

Spicy Sesame Prawn
Noodle Salad
(see page 218)

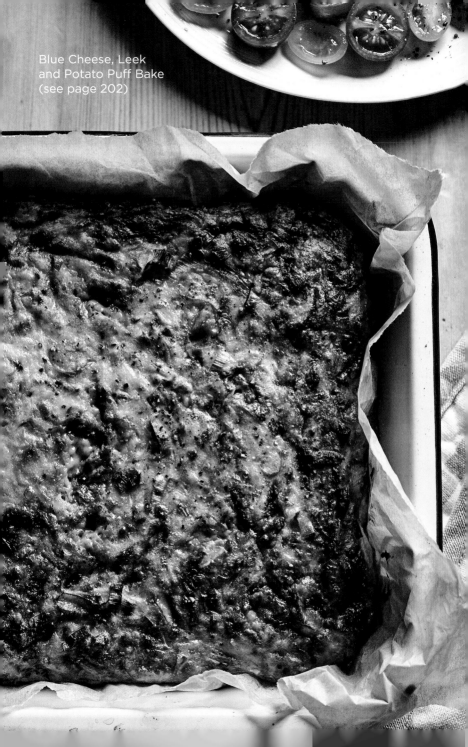

Blue Cheese, Leek
and Potato Puff Bake
(see page 202)

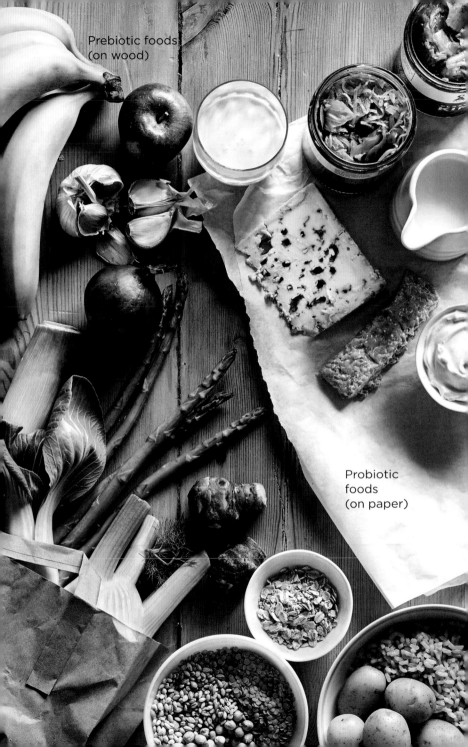

Prebiotic foods
(on wood)

Probiotic
foods
(on paper)

Heart-Warmer Porridge with Banana, Cinnamon and Pecans

306 calories, 7g protein, 1 portion fruit

Does exactly what it says: warms you up and sets you up for the day.
See over for lots of other variations that are just as nurturing!

Serves 1
Preparation time: 5 minutes
Cooking time: 5 minutes

100ml skimmed dairy or almond milk

40g jumbo oats

½ tsp ground cinnamon

Pinch of salt

For the banana topping:

2 teaspoons maple syrup

1 small banana, 80g without skin, cut into pieces

7g unsalted pecans, finely chopped or crushed OR 1 tsp ground flaxseeds/mixed seeds

To serve:

Pinch of ground cinnamon, for dusting

1. Put the milk and 150ml water in a medium saucepan and add the oats. Heat gently until just below boiling. Turn the heat down to low.
2. Add the cinnamon and salt and cook for 5 minutes, making sure the mix doesn't stick to the pan. (You can

also microwave the oats, liquid, cinnamon and salt in a large, partly covered bowl: do it 30 seconds at a time, and watch closely as it's very prone to boiling over. It takes 2–3 minutes.) Let it stand for 2 minutes before eating.

3. Serve the porridge with the fruit and syrup mixed through, and sprinkle with the nuts or seeds.

VARIATIONS: Use a few drops of vanilla or almond extract while cooking the porridge, or add half a teaspoon of unsweetened cocoa powder. Use any favourite fruits as a topping.

PLENTY DAY SUGGESTIONS: It's lovely with Greek yogurt or extra nuts on the topping.

Mexican Tomato Scramble on Toast.
Vegan version

308 calories, 19g protein; vegetarian version: 318 calories, 17g protein.

Both 1 portion of veg

Spicy and a great wake-up kick. Of course, you can just scramble the eggs or tofu, but this adds a little veg to your morning meal!

Serves 1

Preparation time: 3 minutes

Cooking time: 4–6 minutes

100g firm plain tofu or 2 medium eggs

1 tsp oil or butter

6 cherry tomatoes, finely chopped

½–1 tsp chipotle paste or 1 small chipotle pepper rehydrated in a little water and finely chopped

¼ tsp ground cumin

¼ tsp dried thyme

1 spring onion, chopped (optional)

1 x 50g slice of sourdough bread

To serve:

Fresh coriander

1. If using eggs, break them into a mug and beat lightly with a fork. For the tofu, drain from the packet and use kitchen roll to press out as much moisture as you can. Break up with a fork.

2. Heat the oil or butter in a small non-stick saucepan. Add the tomatoes, chipotle, cumin, thyme and spring onion if using and fry over a high heat for 2 minutes. Now lower the heat and add the eggs or tofu. For the eggs, move them around the pan as the egg sets, until they reach the texture you like (remember they carry on cooking once you've turned off the heat). For the tofu, sauté until the edges are lightly browned.
3. Toast the bread, top with the scramble, and garnish with fresh coriander.

VARIATIONS: Scramble with 25g baby spinach instead of – or as well as – the tomatoes.

PLENTY DAY SUGGESTIONS: Add an extra egg, or more tofu, or serve with mashed or sliced avocado or black beans on the side. Non-veggies can add 25g chorizo or bacon to the pan with the spices and tomatoes.

Soups and light meals

Packed with flavour, not calories – all the recipes in this section make a great lunch or light supper. They're also really useful as starters if you're planning a single big meal on a Fast Day, or to introduce friends to the joys of the Dirty Diet!

Mexican Smoky Bean Soup with Kefir Swirl

142 calories, 7g protein, 3 servings of veg

This is a brilliant store-cupboard soup as it's mainly made from tins of beans and veg. But it tastes fresh and zingy thanks to the lime and the kefir, and you can make it super fast. Freezes so well too!

Makes 4 servings
Preparation time: 5 minutes
Cooking time: 6 minutes

1 tsp extra-virgin olive oil
1 medium red onion, chopped
1 medium yellow pepper, cut into pieces
1 tsp cumin
10g/2 tsp chipotle chilli paste
½–1 tsp chilli powder
1 x 400g tin chopped tomatoes
300–500ml vegetable stock, home-made or made with
2 tsp vegetable bouillon powder
1 x 400g can mixed beans in water, drained
100g sweetcorn kernels, frozen or tinned
Juice of ½ lime

To serve:
60g dairy or coconut kefir
Fresh coriander leaves

1. Heat the oil and fry the onion, yellow pepper, cumin, chipotle paste and chilli powder together in a large saucepan for 3 minutes.
2. Add the tinned tomatoes, stock, beans and sweetcorn. Heat through for another 3 minutes.
3. Squeeze the lime into the soup and, if you like, use a hand blender to blend some of the beans and vegetables for a thicker texture.
4. Season, and serve with kefir swirled through and the coriander on top.

VARIATIONS: Use whichever beans you have to hand – black or pinto beans work well.

PLENTY DAY SUGGESTIONS: Serve with a slice of Avocado Toast from the breakfast recipes (p. 158).

Green Star Minestrone with Pesto

153 calories, 9g protein; non-vegetarian version: 188 calories, 11g protein. Both 2 portions of veg.

A super-satisfying and beautiful soup for summer or winter – the pesto brings the other flavours to life, though you need to use it sparingly. Do chop the vegetables really small to make the soup look as good as it tastes.

Makes 4 servings
Preparation time: 20 minutes
Cooking time: 10–14 minutes

1 tsp olive oil
1 small onion, peeled and finely chopped
2 celery sticks, finely chopped
1 courgette (170g), finely diced
2 garlic cloves, finely chopped
1 litre stock made with 3 tsp vegetable bouillon powder or good-quality chicken stock cube
100g green beans, trimmed and chopped into small pieces
1 x 400g can borlotti or cannellini beans, drained
30g tiny pasta shapes, e.g. stellette or orzo
80g baby spinach
2 tsp fresh basil pesto
15g finely grated Parmesan or Grana Padano or veggie Italian cheese
40g pancetta (optional)

1. Warm the olive oil in a large saucepan. Add the onion, celery, courgette, and pancetta if using. Gently fry over a low heat for 3–4 minutes or until softened but not coloured. Add the garlic and fry for a further minute.
2. Add the hot stock, green and tinned beans and the little pasta shapes. Bring to the boil and simmer for 4–7 minutes (check pasta instructions), then add spinach and cook for 1 minute. Taste and season well.
3. To serve, divide the soup between bowls, drizzle with half a teaspoon of pesto each (it *is* high in calories) and scatter with the grated cheese.

PLENTY DAY SUGGESTION: enjoy with a slice of sourdough toast rubbed with garlic after toasting.

Chickpea and Leek Soup with Blue Cheese

144 calories (or 170 calories if made with potatoes) 8.4g protein,

2 portions of veg

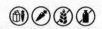

This is so hearty and savoury – and it's going to get your friendly bacteria doing the happy dance too, with a mix of prebiotic food from the leeks, garlic and chickpeas, plus the probiotic blue cheese. Super fast, too.

Makes 4 servings

Preparation time: 5 minutes

Cooking time: 10 minutes (with tinned beans)

1 x 400g tin chickpeas, drained, or 75g uncooked

5g butter or oil

2 medium leeks, around 200g, chopped

200g celeriac or pre-cooked new potatoes, grated

½ tsp dried thyme

2 garlic cloves

900ml vegetable stock, home-made or made from 2 tsp vegetable bouillon powder

To serve:

40g blue cheese topping (10g per bowl)

(Or use seeds for a vegan soup)

1. If using dried chickpeas, soak them in cold water overnight. Rinse and drain the next morning.

2. Heat the butter or oil in a large saucepan and gently fry the leeks and celeriac or potatoes for 3 minutes, stirring to ensure they don't burn. Add the thyme, chickpeas, garlic and stock and bring to the boil. If using tinned chickpeas, cook for another 5 minutes or so. If using soaked dried chickpeas, simmer for an hour, making sure to top up the water now and then to ensure it doesn't boil dry. Check the chickpeas are cooked – it'll take around 1 hour 15–30 minutes.
3. If you like a smooth soup, use a stick blender to blend once the beans are cooked or warmed through.
4. Season and serve, crumbling the blue cheese over the top to melt (or top with seeds).

VARIATIONS: It's also tasty with a little pesto, or Grana Padano grated on top, in place of the blue cheese.

The soup freezes well. Don't add the cheese before freezing, but after re-heating.

Tomato and Strawberry Gazpacho

With egg: 145 calories, 6.2g protein; with sunflower seeds: 150 calories,
4.3g protein. Both 3 portions of fruit and veg

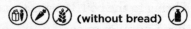 **(without bread)**

This is the perfect summer recipe! Chilled soup sometimes freaks people out, but it shouldn't. Imagine a cross between a refreshing salad and a cooling drink – with lots of fresh veg and a satisfying kick. Give it a whirl. In Spain, it's common to use fruits (a tomato is a fruit, after all), and strawberries give a perfect sweet-sour flavour, while the optional bread adds a thicker texture.

Makes 4 servings
Preparation time: 10 minutes

1 small bread roll or 60g sliced stale sourdough bread
(optional)
600g deep red, ripe tomatoes, chopped
1 large garlic clove, chopped
1 red pepper, chopped
½ large cucumber (125g)
75g ripe strawberries
2 tbsp sherry vinegar
1 tbsp olive oil

For the garnish:
2 strawberries, halved
4 cherry tomatoes, halved
2 hard-boiled eggs (chopped) or 25g sunflower seeds

1. Soak the bread in a little water (if using). Roughly chop the garlic, vegetables and fruit and then blend or food process till smooth. Add the bread, if using, and blend again. Taste, season and add vinegar and oil. Blend a last time.
2. Either chill or serve at room temperature. Garnish with the strawberries and cherry tomatoes plus chopped egg or sunflower seeds.

VARIATIONS: Serve with croutons: for 4 servings, fry cubes of 2 thick slices of sourdough or seeded bread in a small frying pan in 2 tsp oil over a medium heat until golden. Adds 80 calories per serving.

Try 1 juicy kiwi fruit in place of the strawberries – if you can get the golden fruit or, best of all, the tiny grape ones that don't need peeling; even better. Taste before adding the vinegar as kiwis can be quite tart. The calorie count is the same.

Pumpkin and Lentil Soup with Herb-Infused Olive Oil

153 calories, 5.4g protein, 2 portions of veg

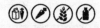

Red lentils are so quick and filling and, combined with the pumpkin or squash, give this autumnal soup a lovely colour and texture. The quantities of herb oil are small (to keep calories lower) but it really packs a flavour punch.

Makes 4 servings
Preparation time: 5 minutes
Cooking time: 20 minutes

15ml oil
1 onion, chopped
400g pumpkin flesh or butternut squash, cubed
75g red lentils
2-inch-piece fresh ginger, grated
500ml vegetable or chicken stock, home-made or from vegetable bouillon power
1 tsp dried or fresh, chopped woody herbs, e.g. rosemary, thyme
1 garlic clove, crushed

1. Heat ½ teaspoon of the oil in a large non-stick saucepan and fry the onion for 2–3 minutes till soft.
2. Add the pumpkin, red lentils, ginger and stock plus 200ml water to the pan and turn up the heat to bring to the boil.

Turn down the heat and simmer for 20 minutes, till the lentils have cooked and the pumpkin or squash is soft.

3. Meanwhile, make the oil. Add the remaining oil to a very small frying pan or place in a small dish. Add the herbs and heat gently for a couple of minutes. Remove from heat and stir in the crushed garlic (this ensures it won't burn).

4. Purée with a hand blender, adding enough water to bring it to your preferred texture for 4 portions.

5. Serve the soup with ½ teaspoon of the oil, drizzled on top and stirred through.

How to invent your own easy, delicious soup recipe

There's no big secret to delicious soup – this is the basic method I use when I am planning to make one. You can calorie count quite easily, and this makes 3–4 portions. Keep covered in the fridge for up to 3 days, or freeze in individual portions.

You need:

1 saucepan

1 hand blender (if you want to purée the soup)

1 tsp fat: olive oil, rapeseed oil, butter or coconut oil

1 onion or a stick of celery, chopped

Fresh flavourings: try chopped garlic, a fresh chilli, chopped (wash your hands afterwards!)

Herbs and spices: choose your favourites from the spice rack or the garden: around 1 teaspoon of dried spices or a small handful of fresh herb leaves will add lots of flavour – stick to one or two different flavours until you're feeling confident. Add whole spices and bay leaves, dried herbs, rosemary or thyme to the cooking pot. Fresh mint, parsley, basil and coriander are best added just before serving or as a garnish.

400g vegetables: use seasonal produce or frozen veg like peas (delicious with mint) or carrots. Aim for 2–3 varieties that you like together.

75g leaves: baby spinach, kale, chard, spring greens. Wash well and remove any very thick stems. Chop roughly if the leaves are not baby leaves.

Store cupboard extras: a can of chopped Italian tomatoes or a drained can of cooked lentils or beans will add body and flavour.

750ml stock: use vegetable bouillon powder or chicken stock cubes.

Your choice of toppings: fresh herbs, grated cheese like Cheddar or Parmesan, a spoonful of Greek yogurt or crème fraîche, a sprinkling of seeds or a dash of hot chilli sauce.

1. Heat the fat in the saucepan and add the onion or celery with any dried herbs or spices or spice pastes and cook gently for 5 minutes till the vegetables are translucent. Meanwhile, chop root veg like potatoes or carrots into cubes and slice green vegetables.

2. Add the vegetables to the pan along with any woody fresh herbs like thyme or rosemary and let them cook – root vegetables benefit from browning a tad. Now add the stock and bring to the boil.

3. Let the soup simmer until the toughest vegetables are just soft – for carrots or potatoes, this might take 20–25 minutes, for green beans or cauliflower, much less.

4. Add leaves, if using, and let them wilt for 2–3 minutes. Purée the soup using a hand blender if you wish. Season with black pepper and sea salt. Serve with your choice of toppings and a chunk of good bread.

MY FAVOURITE EASY COMBINATIONS

Carrot and coriander: 400g carrots, 1 onion, 1 clove garlic, 1 tsp ground coriander, 75g spinach. To serve: 1 tbsp yogurt, with fresh parsley or fresh coriander on top.

Sweet potato and chilli: 400g sweet potatoes, peeled, 1 red onion, 75g baby kale or greens, 1 fresh chilli, 1 tsp ground cumin or curry powder/garam masala. To serve: a little chilli sauce and some fresh chives.

Cauliflower cheese: 1 small head of cauliflower divided into florets, 1 onion or leek, 1 small potato, diced, 1 tsp wholegrain mustard. To serve: grated Cheddar cheese over the top and, if you like it, add some fresh young rocket leaves for a peppery flavour.

Quick-as-a-Flash Cauliflower and Broccoli Tabbouleh

131 calories, 7g protein, 3 portions of veg

This is one of those dishes that has it all – it's high in veg, it's so fast to make and it looks gorgeous. It tastes fresh and delicious and keeps for a day in the fridge so you can take it to work as well. You do need a food processor, a mini chopper or good knife skills though! I use one of those small packs of cauliflower and broccoli florets as a cheat . . .

Serves 2

Preparation time: 5 minutes

200g mixed cauliflower and broccoli florets

Handful fresh mint

Handful fresh parsley

3 spring onions, roughly chopped

30g fresh pomegranate seeds

150g cherry tomatoes, halved

Juice of 1 lemon

1 tsp extra-virgin olive oil

10g sunflower or pumpkin seeds

1. Pulse the florets in a food processor or chopper till they form 'grains' or grate using a cheese grater. Turn out onto a serving plate.

2. Now pulse the herbs and spring onions together, or chop very finely by hand. Reserve a few herbs for the garnish.
3. Mix the chopped herbs with the vegetable 'grains'. Scatter the pomegranate seeds, tomatoes and reserved herbs on top. Pour over the lemon juice and oil, sprinkle with the seeds, and serve.

VARIATIONS: For a slightly nuttier flavour, brown the vegetable 'grains' and seeds. After processing, but before adding the herbs, pat the cauliflower and broccoli dry with kitchen roll. Heat an extra ½ teaspoon of oil (21 calories) in a large pan and fry the 'grains' over a high heat till they start to brown a little. Remove from the pan onto the serving dish. Brown the sunflower seeds in the same pan. Continue with the recipe as above.

PLENTY DAY OPTIONS: Serve with falafel or sliced grilled halloumi cheese.

Hot Artichoke and Pepper Spread with Mozzarella on Sourdough Toast

137 calories, 7.5g protein, 1 portion of veg

Artichokes are great for gut health but they're fussy to prepare – tinned ones are cheaper and are so easy. I use a stick blender to whizz it all together, which means minimal washing up! This works as a cold dip too.

Serves 4
Preparation time: 8 minutes
Cooking time: 3–4 minutes

1 x 390g tin artichoke hearts, drained and rinsed
Juice of 1 lemon
1 garlic clove, roughly chopped
20g sun-dried tomatoes, oil drained off
2 medium yellow or red bell peppers, roughly chopped
½ ball light mozzarella cheese
4 x 30g slices (very thinly cut) sourdough bread

1. Heat the grill to medium. Add all the ingredients except the cheese and bread to the hand blender container and combine well. Season to taste.
2. Toast the bread lightly on both sides then spread each slice with a quarter of the spread. Cut the mozzarella into very thin slices and place on the top. Grill for 2–3 minutes until the mix is warm and the cheese is starting to brown.

189

VARIATIONS: Try with capers and spring onions in the spread instead of the pepper. Also tasty without the cheese.

PLENTY DAY SUGGESTION: This is really delicious served with soup for a light lunch.

Egg Pancake with Quick-Blistered Veg

147 calories, 10g protein, 1.5 portions of veg

This is my go-to lunch if I am in a hurry and short on ideas – I just improvise with whatever veg is in the fridge and whichever spices I fancy. The pancake is also really satisfying thanks to the mix of protein and fibre.

Serves 1

Preparation time: 5 minutes

Cooking time: 4 minutes

1 tsp sesame oil, rapeseed oil, olive oil, coconut oil or butter

120g mixed mangetout/baby corn or other stir-fry vegetables

Soy sauce or tamari sauce (optional)

1 tsp whole seeds, e.g. coriander, onion seed

1 medium egg

1. First, heat half the oil or butter to a high temperature in a small non-stick pan, e.g. an omelette pan. Cook the vegetables, letting them brown slightly. Add a little soy sauce or tamari sauce if you like. Set aside.
2. Add second half of the oil and toast the seeds. Break the egg into a mug or bowl, beat lightly, then season and pour into the hot pan – tilt to cover the surface thinly.

3. Cook for 1–2 minutes then check with a spatula to see when it's brown underneath. If so, flip it over and cook for a further 1–2 minutes. Serve topped with the vegetables.

VARIATIONS: Use fermented veg as a crunchy filling e.g. the home-made fresh apple and red cabbage sauerkraut from p. 295. Chopped chives added to the egg pancake give a lovely subtle onion flavour.

Wedge Salad with Blue Cheese Dressing

120 calories, 6g protein, 2 portions of veg

Iceberg lettuce is traditionally used for a wedge salad but I find it tasteless, and it has very little nutritional value. I prefer to use romaine – with this simple but tangy probiotic dressing and a few crunchy nuts on top. Use strong blue cheese – a little goes a long way!

Serves 1
Preparation time: 3 minutes

10g Roquefort or other blue cheese
35ml kefir
¼– ½ tsp cayenne pepper
5 pistachio nuts
½ romaine lettuce, cut into wedges
6 cherry tomatoes, halved

1. Grate or crumble the blue cheese. Place in a small dish and use a metal spoon to beat together with the kefir and the cayenne. Remove shells from the pistachios and crush gently.
2. Lay the lettuce wedges and tomatoes on a plate, pour over the kefir dressing. Season and sprinkle over the crushed nuts.

VARIATIONS: This also works well with griddled radicchio or red chicory: cut into wedges or quarters, then lightly oil a grill pan and place the lettuces cut side down. Check every 60 seconds during griddling to ensure leaves brown but don't burn. They'll take around 2 minutes.

Pink Tzatziki with Super-Fast Chickpea Flatbread

177 calories, 8g protein, 1 portion of veg

Tasty and nutritious . . . a great savoury way to enjoy yogurt and fresh veg. The beetroot tzatziki is a lovely colour, and the flatbread is so fast. It's like a cross between a pancake and a pizza base – just remember to let the batter stand for a little while before using; you can also keep it in the fridge.

Serves 4
Preparation time: 40 minutes
Cooking time: 7 minutes

For the tzatziki:
125ml Greek yogurt or coconut yogurt
2 tbsp kefir
200g cucumber, finely diced
2 tbsp chopped fresh mint, plus mint sprigs to garnish
1 tsp ground cumin
100g raw beetroot, peeled and grated
1 small garlic clove, crushed
Salt and pepper

For the chickpea flatbread (makes 4):
100g gram flour
½ teaspoon chilli flakes or powder
2 tsp olive oil

1. Mix gram flour, chilli flakes and 200ml water together in a jug, stirring well so there are no lumps. Leave to stand for at least 30 minutes.
2. Meanwhile, make the tzatziki. Beat together the yogurt and kefir, then add the other ingredients and season well with salt and pepper. Spoon into a serving dish and garnish with mint sprigs.
3. Heat a little of the olive oil in a small non-stick omelette pan or frying pan – use a pastry brush to distribute it. Add a quarter of the batter to the pan and cook over a medium heat for 2–3 minutes till cooked underneath. Now flip the pancake, and cook for 2 more minutes
4. Serve warm and spread with the tzatziki, or use as a dip.

VARIATIONS:

Feta and chilli tzatziki: Add 40g of crumbled feta or a lighter salad cheese (adds 65–90 calories, so 17–22 calories per portion) and swirl hot chilli powder instead of cumin into the dip.

Apple tzatziki: Grate 2 small tart dessert apples into the yogurt mix instead of (or as well as) the beetroot. Adds 70 calories, or 18 per portion.

The flatbread works with many different whole or ground spices in the batter. You can also use the flatbread as a pizza base – add pizza toppings after cooking and finish under the grill.

Thyme and Sweet Pepper Hummus
with Crudités

153 calories, 7.2g protein, 3 portions of veg

Hummus is good for you, but the creamier it is, the more oil – or emulsifiers – might have gone into it. So you'll need to add other flavours too if you want to keep calories down. This version is super quick and tasty, and is flavoured with za'atar, a tasty mix of thyme and sesame seeds.

Makes 4 servings
Preparation time: 5 minutes

Juice of 1 lemon

1 yellow or red pepper, roughly chopped

1 x 400g tin chickpeas, drained

2 garlic cloves

15ml/1 tbsp tahini

2 tsp olive oil

2 tsp za'atar (reserve some for gsarnish) or 1 tsp each dried thyme and sesame seeds

Crudités for 4:

150g crisp lettuce leaves, such as little gem

1 medium cucumber, around 100g, cut into sticks

2 medium carrots, cut into batons or sticks

1 red, yellow or green pepper, sliced

1. Blend the lemon juice and pepper first. Then add the chickpeas and the other ingredients. Stir through the za'atar, reserving a little for garnish. Season (but watch the salt, since za'atar can be quite salty).
2. Sprinkle a little za'atar on the top and serve with the crudités.

VARIATION: Use hot harissa paste instead of the za'atar.

PLENTY DAY SUGGESTION: This makes a great filling for four wholemeal pitta breads – each filled pitta is 298 calories and 13g protein, so it also works as a light summery Fast Day lunch or dinner.

Main dishes

These are satisfying and delicious – most of the dishes have a Fast Day version, with suggestions for adding extras for your Plenty Days, or to feed a crowd.

Revved-Up Caesar Salad with Parmesan and Mustard Kefir Dressing

319 calories, 13g protein (chicken version 42g protein),

3 portions of veg

This is super filling and very tasty indeed. Sliced raw asparagus is delicious but, if you prefer, blanch the spears whole in a pan of boiling water for 2 minutes until just tender. The chicken version is higher in protein but is the same calories.

Serves 1

Preparation time: 15 minutes

Cooking time: 10–12 minutes (only if using chicken)

½ medium avocado OR 1 x 130g raw chicken breast

1 small (25g) slice sourdough or seeded wholegrain bread, cut into cubes

3 spears of asparagus

40g drained tinned cannellini beans

½ ruby gem lettuce, separated into leaves and torn

¼ cucumber, sliced

For the dressing:

10g Parmesan or veggie Italian cheese, finely grated

2 tbsp kefir

1 tsp white wine vinegar

1 tsp wholegrain mustard

1. If using chicken, preheat the grill to medium. Thickly slice the chicken, place on a baking sheet and season. Grill for 10–12 minutes, or until golden, then turn over and cook the other side. Cut one of the thicker slices in half to check it's cooked. There should be no pink juices or fleshy parts inside. Place the chicken in a large bowl.
2. If using avocado, cut into cubes. (Save the other half of the avocado by keeping the stone in, dropping lemon juice onto the flesh, and storing in the fridge, or cover with cling film.)
3. Add the bread cubes to the baking sheet and grill until golden on both sides, then add to the avocado/chicken in the bowl.
4. Slice the asparagus diagonally along the stalk, or use a vegetable peeler to create thick shavings. Put in the bowl with the avocado/chicken, beans and bread, then add the lettuce and cucumber.
5. Mix together the Parmesan, kefir, vinegar and mustard and season with black pepper. Drizzle the dressing over the salad to serve.

PLENTY DAY SUGGESTIONS: Use both chicken and avocado for a dish that is 457 calories with 56g protein: fantastic for after a workout.

Blue Cheese, Leek and Potato Puff Bake

274 calories, 18g protein, 1 portion of veg

This is light and delicious, with a strong savoury tang of blue cheese. The pre-cooked potatoes are high in resistant starch, making them a feast for your gut bacteria, yet it puffs up beautifully and is also super adaptable. You can use other cheeses or add herbs or spices to change the flavour. It tastes good cold as well as warm, and keeps for a couple of days in the fridge.

Serves 4

Preparation time: 10 minutes

Cooking time: 30–35 minutes (plus parboiling the potatoes in advance, 10–15 minutes)

1 tsp butter or oil

2 medium leeks (200g) shredded

2 spring onions, shredded

200g new potatoes, parboiled till tender and allowed to cool

1 tbsp plain flour

2 tsp baking powder

6 eggs

1 tbsp Greek yogurt

100g blue cheese

1 tsp sea salt flakes

1. Preheat the oven to 200°C/180°C fan/400°F/Gas mark 6. Line a 7 inch/18cm square baking tin with non-stick paper.
2. Sauté the leeks and spring onions for 10 minutes and set aside. Grate the potatoes.
3. Mix the potatoes, flour and baking powder together in a large bowl. Beat the eggs well in another bowl or cup, then add to the dry ingredients. Mix in the cooked leeks and onions, followed by the yogurt and two-thirds of the blue cheese. Season.
4. Pour the mixture into the prepared tin. Sprinkle over the last of the blue cheese.
5. Bake for 20–25 minutes till brown and puffed up.
6. Cut and serve warm or cold with a tomato salad.

VARIATION: replace leeks with steamed fine asparagus and the blue cheese with goat's cheese for a light springtime version with similar calories.

5-a-Day Vegetable and Paneer Balti

297 calories, 20g protein, 5 portions of veg

This is one of those win-win dishes: quick to make, spicy, some tasty protein from the cheese (or tofu), and five different veggie portions. Plus the second portion will keep covered in the fridge for a day or two.

Serves 2
Preparation time: 5 minutes
Cooking time: 10–14 minutes

1 tsp olive oil or coconut oil

125g paneer (I use Apetina which is slightly lower in fat than some paneer but very tasty), cubed OR 150g plain tofu

50g balti spice paste from a jar

1 medium red onion, sliced

1 small red chilli pepper, chopped, seeds and membrane removed

1 green pepper, sliced

200g cauliflower, broken into florets

200g raw tomatoes or passata

1 garlic clove, crushed or chopped

100g green or French beans, sliced diagonally

To serve:
Fresh coriander leaves

1. In a large saucepan, gently fry the paneer in the oil and 1 teaspoon of the balti paste, until the edges are browned: around 2–3 minutes. Set aside on a plate.
2. Add the rest of the paste to the same pan, and fry the onion, chilli, sliced pepper and cauliflower florets for 3–4 minutes: add a little water if the vegetables start to burn rather than brown. Now add the tomatoes, crushed garlic, green beans and a little water to cover. Cook till the cauliflower is just tender, around 5–6 minutes, adding extra water if needed. Stir the cooked paneer back into the balti to warm through again.
3. Serve garnished with fresh coriander.

PLENTY DAY SUGGESTIONS: serve with brown basmati rice or a heated chapatti.

Chicken Dirty Rice with Spices and Bacon

345 calories, 21g protein, 2.5 portions of veg

Well, this is the Dirty Diet book, so dirty rice definitely belongs. It's an ideal supper dish for two people, but you can also keep one portion in the fridge for the next day (but ensure it's chilled straight away and then served piping hot because rice can sometimes cause food poisoning). This dish is an adaptation of a Cajun dish. The traditional version involves chicken livers and pork but this simpler one uses lower-fat chicken sausages, and lardons for flavour (you could also use pork sausages). Really filling and tasty! And there's a veggie version too, with a little less rice, and more pulses.

Serves 2

Preparation time: 10 minutes

Cooking time: 14 minutes (plus 20–25 minutes for the rice)

100g wholegrain basmati rice

5g butter or oil

1 red onion, finely chopped

1 large celery stick, chopped

1 green pepper

1 yellow pepper

4 lower-fat chicken chipolatas, e.g. Heck, cut into chunks

25g smoked bacon lardons

1 tsp Cajun seasoning OR ¼ tsp each paprika, cayenne, dried oregano and dried thyme

To serve:

Fresh parsley or thyme, chopped

1. Cook the rice – rinse and then cover with cold water, bring to the boil and simmer for 20–25 minutes, topping up with water if needed (or use a microwaveable sachet if you're in a hurry).
2. Heat the oil in a large non-stick pan and add the onion, celery, peppers, chicken, bacon and the Cajun seasoning. Cook over medium heat for 12 minutes (or according to sausage pack instructions). Let the meat brown in places – it'll give the rice colour and flavour.
3. Add the rice and cook together over a medium heat for another minute or two, so the rice is lightly fried and warmed through. Serve garnished with fresh parsley or thyme.

Veggie Dirty Rice with Spices and Sausages

324 calories, 13g protein, 2 portions veg

Serves 2

Preparation time: 10 minutes

Cooking time: 10 minutes (plus 20–25 minutes for the rice)

80g wholegrain basmati rice

5g butter or oil

1 red onion, finely chopped

1 large celery stick, chopped

1 green pepper

½ yellow pepper

2 veggie sausages

1 tsp Cajun seasoning OR ¼ tsp each paprika, cayenne, dried oregano and dried thyme

100g precooked Puy lentils or other pulses

• Cook as for Chicken Dirty Rice, but add the Puy lentils at the same time as the rice to warm through.

Mushroom and Tofu/Chicken Stroganoff

Tofu version: 303 calories

Chicken version: 302 calories, 34g protein. Both: 3 portions of veg

A version of this dish was in my very first 5:2 book, but I went back to basics for this new, richer, even more filling version. Mushrooms are centre-stage, followed by paprika, leeks and a creamy sauce. The order of cooking seems fiddly but it is easier than it sounds and gives the best results.

Serves 2
Preparation time: 5 minutes
Cooking time: 15 minutes

6g dried mushrooms
200g plain tofu (or 220g diced chicken breast)
2 tsp butter or olive oil
1 tsp sweet or smoked paprika, plus extra for sprinkling
1 small red onion, diced
2 large leeks, chopped
250g mixed mushrooms, chopped or sliced (use your favourite variety, but chestnut and shiitake together work well in this dish)
Squeeze lemon juice
1 garlic clove, chopped or crushed
70g reduced-fat crème fraîche OR coconut yogurt

To serve:
Fresh parsley or chives, chopped

209

1. Soak the dried mushrooms in 50ml boiling water for at least 10 minutes while you cook the other vegetables.
2. Drain the tofu and pat dry with kitchen roll, then dice.
3. Heat 1 teaspoon of butter or oil with ½ teaspoon paprika in a large non-stick frying pan. Fry the tofu cubes till they firm up, then set them aside on a plate. If using chicken, fry until cooked through, around 5–6 minutes depending on the size of the pieces, then set aside.
4. Heat the second teaspoon of oil/butter in same pan, and cook the onion and leeks for 3 minutes. Add to the plate with the tofu/chicken.
5. Add the mushrooms to the empty pan with the other ½ teaspoon of paprika and a squeeze of lemon juice (this helps prevent the mushrooms from sticking to the pan). Turn up the heat and cook till the edges of the mushrooms start to catch, around 4–5 minutes.
6. Tip the soaked mushrooms plus the liquid into the pan with the garlic, and add the tofu/chicken, onions and leeks. Heat through, using the spatula to loosen any caramelised mushroom from the pan to add to the flavour.
7. Remove the pan from the heat and stir in the crème fraîche, mixing well. Season with salt and pepper. Serve topped with chopped parsley or chives and a sprinkling of paprika.

PLENTY DAY SUGGESTIONS: serve with wholegrain basmati rice or with sourdough toast, rubbed with the cut side of half a clove of garlic for super-fast garlic bread.

Middle Eastern Spiced Bean Burgers with Halloumi and Aubergine 'Buns'

310 calories, 19g protein, 3 portions of veg

Making a good home-made veggie burger can be quite a challenge: they need bags of flavour, and the right colour and texture. These deliver. They may have more ingredients than most, but they freeze really well and are great to have on standby. The aubergine 'buns' add another veg and fit with the middle-eastern theme, but when it's not a Fast Day, feel free to use a sourdough bun.

Serves 4

Preparation time: 15 minutes

Cooking time: 10 minutes to fry, 20–25 minutes to bake

4 spring onions, snipped

2 tsp Moroccan-style seasoning or ½ teaspoon ground cumin plus ¼ teaspoon each of ground ginger, ground cinnamon and ground coriander

1 x 400g can mixed beans in water, drained and rinsed

1 handful fresh coriander leaves

1 handful fresh mint

100g beetroot, raw, peeled

50g jumbo rolled oats (or panko breadcrumbs)

1 medium egg

75g light feta cheese or smoked tofu, cubed or crumbled

1 tbsp olive oil (if baking) or 15ml olive oil (if frying)

To serve:

1 medium aubergine (300g)

1 tsp olive oil

100g reduced-fat halloumi, thinly sliced, or smoked tofu

40g reduced-fat hummus, or spicy relish

4 slices (68g) tomatoes, raw

50g pea shoots or rocket

12 cherry tomatoes

1. Combine the onions, seasoning, beans, herbs, beetroot and rolled oats in a food processor. Beat the egg and add half at first then check the consistency – it will be loose but still capable of shaping into patties. Add more egg as needed to reach the right consistency. Finally, stir in the crumbled cheese or tofu.

2. Place the mixture in a bowl and put in the fridge to chill for at least 20 minutes to make the burgers easier to shape (you can leave them for up to a day before cooking). When you want to shape the burgers, wet your hands lightly, then divide the mixture roughly into four and create two burgers from each quarter (i.e. you end up with 8 burgers).

3. To make the aubergine buns and halloumi/tofu, cut the aubergine into 8 rounds around 1cm deep (discard the narrower top or use in roasted veg). Using a pastry brush, brush lightly with the remaining teaspoon of olive oil and place oiled side down in a non-stick pan or griddle. Cook over a high heat for about 4 minutes till they start to brown, then brush topside with oil and turn to cook the other side. Place on kitchen roll while you dry-fry the

halloumi or tofu pieces till they're brown on both sides.

4. When the burgers are ready to cook, either place 2 burgers per serving on a baking sheet and brush lightly with the oil, then bake in the oven at 200°C/180°C fan/400°F/Gas mark 6 for 25 minutes, turning once or fry in a saucepan in olive oil till golden brown, around 5 minutes on each side.

5. To assemble, place one burger on top of one round of aubergine, add the halloumi or tofu, then the second burger, then the hummus or relish, a slice of tomato and some pea shoots/rocket, then top with a second aubergine round and serve with the remaining salad.

How to freeze: Place the uncooked burgers on a baking sheet lined with non-stick baking paper. Freeze until they are solid, then pack into a freezer-proof plastic container and freeze for up to 3 months. You can cook the burgers from frozen: preheat the oven to 200°C/180°C fan/400°F/Gas mark 6 and preheat a baking sheet. Place the burgers on the lined baking sheet and brush with olive oil. Cook for around 30–35 minutes till piping hot in the centre.

VARIATIONS: You can use any tinned beans for this, with your choice of spicing – try blue cheese, cooked leeks and cannellini beans with Italian dried herbs. If you've pre-grilled the aubergines, you can reheat them in a dry non-stick pan, or in the microwave for 20 seconds.

PLENTY DAY SUGGESTIONS: Serve in sourdough buns with sweet potato wedges and double up on grilled halloumi.

Black Lentil Dal with Tomatoes and Creamy Kefir

276 calories, 18g protein, 1.5 portions veg

There's a fantastic Gujarati restaurant around the corner from me – I interviewed the owner and asked him what his favourite dish was and, to my surprise, he said dal makhani, a simple bowl of dark curried dal, with cream swirled through to give richness. This version is less rich, with kefir instead of double cream, but works well. Soak these little powerhouses overnight to speed up cooking time – though it's still a fairly slow process as they have a denser skin and texture than red split peas.

Serves 4

Preparation Time: 5 minutes (plus overnight soaking)

Cooking Time: 35–45 minutes

250g urad dal black lentils

5g butter or coconut oil

1 medium red onion (150g), finely chopped

1 small fresh red chilli, finely chopped

2–3 cardamom pods, lightly crushed

1 tsp ground turmeric

1 tsp ground cumin

300g cherry tomatoes, roughly chopped

1-inch-piece fresh ginger, grated

2 garlic cloves, crushed

To serve:
100ml dairy or coconut kefir (or use natural yogurt)
Fresh coriander leaves

1. Rinse the lentils well and soak in cold water, ideally overnight.
2. Heat the butter or oil and fry the onion and chilli with the spices but not the ginger or garlic. Add the lentils and 600ml water, bring to the boil and boil for 10 minutes. Lower to a simmer and cook for another 20 minutes, before adding the tomatoes, ginger and garlic.
3. Allow to cook down for another 10 minutes, or more depending on how soft you like your lentils – unlike split red lentils, these won't ever break down to a purée, but can be served as you like them.
4. Just before serving, swirl 25ml per serving of kefir through the dal and top with fresh coriander.

You can freeze this in individual portions – without adding the kefir – and microwave from frozen for instant comfort food.

PLENTY DAY SUGGESTIONS: Serve with basmati rice or an Indian bread/chapatti, salad or yogurt. A fried egg on top is also delicious.

Sweet Potato and Broad Bean Tortilla

293 calories, 16g protein, 1 portion of veg

This is a colourful and filling version of a Spanish omelette, cooked in an omelette pan and then cut into delicious wedges. I like to use frozen baby broad beans as their skins are thinner and less indigestible, or you could use fresh and shell them.

Serves 4

Preparation time: 5 minutes

Cooking time: 21–25 minutes (plus 5 minutes for potatoes if not parboiled)

1 medium sweet potato, peeled (250g), cut into thin slices lengthwise

25ml olive oil

1 tsp smoked paprika

1 red onion, thinly sliced

140g frozen baby broad beans

6 eggs

80g light cottage cheese

1. Boil the sweet potato for 5 minutes till just tender. Drain.
2. Heat 1 teaspoon of the oil in a non-stick omelette pan, and gently fry the sweet potato slices, half the paprika and the onion together for 4-5 minutes until they're softening and caramelising. Tip onto a plate. Meanwhile, cook the broad

beans according to instructions, drain, and add to the potato mix.

3. Beat the eggs and add half the cottage cheese and the rest of the paprika. Season.

4. Add 2 teaspoons of oil to the omelette pan and heat gently. Arrange the cooked sweet potato, beans and onions evenly across the pan. Now pour the beaten eggs over the veg, tipping the pan so the egg runs between the potato slices. Sprinkle the remaining cheese on top, and cook over a medium-high heat for 5–7 minutes, until the bottom of the omelette is brown but not burned and the egg mixture is more set.

5. Place a plate that's larger than the frying pan over the pan and turn the pan upside down, so the uncooked side of the tortilla ends up face-down on the plate. Add the rest of the olive oil to the pan and slide the uncooked side of the omelette onto the bottom of the pan and cook for 4–5 minutes. Alternatively, if your pan is heatproof you can finish the top off under the grill. If you're going to be eating this all hot, it's nice to leave the eggs in the centre slightly runnier. Otherwise cook till firmly set.

6. Cut into 4 wedges. Eat hot or cold with a salad of baby spinach or kale.

PLENTY DAY SUGGESTIONS: Add 50g chopped ham or chorizo at step 2. This is also lovely with some roast vegetables or the Romesco Sauce on p. 261.

Spicy Sesame Prawn Noodle Salad

342 calories, 24.5g protein, 3 portions of veg

*Super-speedy and very tasty: one of our test panel's favourite dishes!
Easy to adapt for vegans (see below). I set a challenge for myself to
prep the veg in the 3 minutes while the noodles are cooking – and I
usually make it! Use more chilli if you like it spicy.*

Serves 1
Preparation time: 7 minutes
Cooking time: 3 minutes

5ml tahini (or you can use runny peanut butter)

5ml soy sauce

5ml fish sauce (or double up on soy)

5ml sesame oil

5ml sweet chilli sauce

1 small chilli, finely chopped

½ shallot, finely chopped

30g thin rice noodles, uncooked

60g baby corn

60g mangetout peas

½ yellow pepper, cut into thin strips

100g cooked, peeled prawns

Handful fresh mint or coriander

½ tsp toasted sesame seeds

1. Mix together the tahini with the soy sauce, fish sauce (if using), sesame oil, chilli sauce, the chilli and the shallot in the base of a shallow serving bowl.
2. Break up the noodles with your fingers and place in a heatproof bowl, with the baby corn and mangetout. Pour over boiling water and leave the noodles to soften for the time listed on the pack (normally 3 minutes). Drain and run under cold water to stop the cooking. Slice the baby corn diagonally across.
3. Add the noodles, blanched vegetables and the pepper to the serving bowl, and use a fork to mix and cover with the dressing. Add the prawns, season, and sprinkle the top with the herbs and seeds.

VARIATIONS: This is also delicious with ready-marinated tofu instead of the prawns – use around 70g for a similar calorie count. I like it with just the veg (270 calories). Or serve warm with a poached or fried egg on top.

Punchy New Potato Salad with Egg and Pea Shoots

284 calories, 15g protein, 2 portions of veg

This is incredibly filling, very portable and so tasty. I love potato salad, and this one replaces gloopy mayo with a sharp olive-oil-and-mustard dressing, which works well with the creamy egg, the herbs and the greens. There's some pre-cooking involved in this, but you can use the same pan – do just allow time for the potatoes to cool down so you get all that gut-friendly resistant starch!

Serves 1
Preparation Time: 10 minutes
Cooking Time: 15–20 minutes

175g new/salad potatoes (e.g. 4 medium Charlottes)

1 medium egg

20g pea shoots

30g baby leaf spinach

80g sugar snap peas, mangetout or French beans

3 spring onions (30g), chopped into rounds, including the green tops

For the dressing:

Small handful of chives

½ tsp Dijon mustard

15ml white wine vinegar

1 tsp extra-virgin olive oil

1. Put the potatoes in a pan with enough water to cover, bring to the boil and simmer for 15–20 minutes, depending on size, until just tender. Remove and allow to cool completely (you can speed this up by placing them in a bowl of cold water.

2. Bring the water back to the boil and lower the egg into the pan. Boil for 30 seconds, then reduce to a simmer and cook for 9–11 minutes, depending on how hard you like your eggs (even 9 minutes will still be solid in the middle). Use a slotted spoon to transfer the egg into a bowl of iced water (that makes it easier to peel once it's cooled down completely).

3. To assemble the salad, make the dressing by whisking together the ingredients or combining in a jar and shaking well.

4. Cut the potatoes into bite-size slices, and place in a serving bowl with the other vegetables: the pea shoots, spinach, peas/beans and spring onions. Pour over the dressing and mix gently.

5. Peel the egg, cut into slices and add to the top of the salad. Serve, or pack in a lunchbox.

VARIATIONS: This is very much a base recipe that works with many different veggie additions, especially if you can find different-coloured produce. I made it with beautiful violet French beans from the garden, it looked amazing. Try replacing the egg with 100g drained tuna chunks in spring water (317 calories in dish) OR 2 slices smoked thin bacon rashers, grilled till crispy and then crumbled (305 calories in dish) – or add both for a Plenty Day meal.

Filo Tart with Brie, Winter Veg and Bacon or Mushrooms

322 calories, 16g protein (or veggie version: 312 calories, 15g protein),

1 portion veg

Who doesn't love a pie on a Fast Day? They're a little fiddly but so pretty. This one has an autumnal flavour, but there's a spring option over as well. You can make this as a large tart too for the family. Work quickly with filo pastry, but don't fret too much if pieces break: the four layers will hold so long as you cook the minute you've added the filling!

Serves 4

Preparation: 10 minutes

Cooking time: 28–35 minutes

25ml extra-virgin olive oil

4 sheets filo pastry

200g leeks, finely sliced

200g mushrooms, sliced

20g smoked bacon lardons (optional)

80g baby kale or spinach, washed

90ml semi-skimmed milk

3 medium eggs

90ml kefir

60g brie, cut into thin slices

You also need 4 individual tart tins or 1 7-inch/20cm loose-bottomed sandwich tin (ideally non-stick) and a pastry brush to apply the oil.

1. Preheat the oven to 200°C/180 °C fan/400°F/Gas mark 6. For individual quiches, cut each sheet into 4 squares. If the tins are non-stick, brush the base and sides with a little oil. Then build up each tart case a sheet of filo at a time, laying them on top of the other, and applying a little oil with the pastry brush for each layer. After adding the fourth layer, crumple the edges down so they're forming a strong 'lip' around the tart. Prebake for 2–5 minutes until the bases and edges are light brown. Remove from the oven and reduce oven temperature to 180°C/160 °C fan/350°F/Gas mark 4.
2. Cook the leeks, mushrooms and bacon (if using) in the remaining oil for 5 minutes. Add the kale to wilt for 1 minute.
3. Beat together milk, eggs and kefir, and season.
4. Spoon the vegetables over the bottom of each quiche. Pour the egg mix over the veg, and arrange the slices of brie on top. Cook immediately, or the base will leak!
5. Bake for 20–22 minutes till set but not rubbery! A large tart will take a little longer.

Springtime Version: Filo Tart with Gruyère, Watercress and Roast Cherry Tomato

315 calories, 16g protein (salmon version: 342 calories, 19g protein),
1 portion of veg

This tasty spring version is delicious with or without the salmon!

Serves 4

Preparation: 10 minutes

Cooking time: 28–35 minutes

150g cherry tomatoes

25ml extra-virgin olive oil

1 red onion

4 sheets filo pastry

60g grated Gruyère cheese

90ml semi-skimmed milk

3 medium eggs

90ml kefir

80g watercress, roughly chopped

Optional: 60g smoked salmon, cut into small pieces

You also need 4 individual tart tins or 1 7-inch/20cm loose-bottomed sandwich tin (ideally non-stick) and a pastry brush to apply the oil.

1. Cut the tomatoes in half, season, and place in a roasting tin – drizzle over 1 teaspoon oil and roast at 200°C/ 180°C fan/400°F/Gas mark 6 for 15 minutes. Slice the

onion finely and add to a separate area of the tin in the last 5 minutes so the slices brown but don't burn. Remove from the oven and set aside.

2. For individual quiches, cut each sheet into 4 squares. If the tins are non-stick, brush the base and sides with a little oil. Then build up each tart case a sheet of filo at a time, laying them on top of the other, and applying a little oil with the pastry brush for each layer. After adding the fourth layer, crumple the edges down so they're forming a strong 'lip' around the tart. Prebake for 2–5 minutes until the bases and edges are light brown. Remove from the oven and reduce oven temperature to 180°C/160 °C fan/350°F/Gas mark 4.

3. Beat together cheese, milk, eggs and kefir, and season: add the salmon if using.

4. Place the watercress and roasted onion on the base of each quiche. Pour over the egg (or egg and salmon) mix, then arrange the cherry tomatoes cut side up on top. Cook immediately, or the base will leak!

5. Bake for 20–22 minutes till set but not rubbery.

Chilli-Spiked Vegetarian Cottage Pie

277 calories, 12.6g protein, 4 portions of veg

This is super hearty and a great source of veg and fibre, from the bright chilli topping to the earthy lentil filling.

Serves 4

Preparation time: 20 minutes

Cooking time: 30 minutes

1 tsp olive or rapeseed oil

1 medium red onion, chopped

2 medium carrots, diced

1 celery stick, chopped

1 tsp paprika or chilli powder

10g dried porcini mushrooms, rehydrated in 50ml water

2 garlic cloves, crushed

1 medium chilli pepper, finely chopped

200g chestnut mushrooms, sliced

1 x 250g pack cooked Puy lentils or drained can of green lentils

200g baby kale or spinach

450g peeled sweet potato

1 heaped tbsp chipotle paste

4 spring onions, chopped

1. Preheat the oven to 200°C/180°C fan/400°F/Gas mark 6. Add the oil to a large non-stick saucepan and fry the onion, carrots and celery with the paprika or chilli powder for 4 minutes.
2. Add the garlic, chilli and chestnut mushrooms and cook for 3 minutes.
3. Add lentils and kale or spinach and the porcini mushrooms, and warm through.
4. Meanwhile, cut the sweet potato into chunks and place in a pan covered with water. Bring to the boil, then simmer till the sweet potato is tender, around 10–15 minutes. Drain well, then mash with the chipotle paste, and mix with spring onions.
5. To assemble the cottage pie, spoon the lentil mixture into a medium ovenproof dish and top with the mash. Bake for 30 minutes, until piping hot.

VARIATIONS: For a more filling version for meat-eaters, add 200g 10% fat minced lamb or beef at the end of stage 1. Let the meat brown, before continuing with stages 2 and 3, then cook on a low heat for 25–30 minutes. Carry on from stage 4. This version is 373 calories with 24g protein.

Beef, Mushroom and Cashew Stir Fry

342 calories, 27g protein, 4–5 portions of veg

This is quick, simple and irresistible – one for people who love steak but want to serve it with a healthy twist. Great for showing to friends or family that 'diet food' is so much more than salads.

Serves 1
Preparation time: 10 minutes (plus time for beef to marinate)
Cooking time: 8 minutes

3 tsp sesame oil or olive oil, reserving 1 tsp
1 medium garlic clove, crushed
15ml soy sauce
1-inch piece fresh ginger, grated
100g stir-fry steak pieces
½ red onion
½ red pepper, finely sliced
3 large leaves Chinese cabbage (145g), shredded
75g shiitake or other exotic mushrooms
To serve:
8g unsalted cashew nut pieces

1. Make the dressing by mixing together half of the sesame oil plus the garlic, soy sauce and ginger in a plastic box. Add the steak pieces, put the lid on and shake well. Ideally, allow to marinate for at least 30 minutes in the fridge.

2. Heat a griddle or wok over a high heat. Cook the steak pieces for 2 minutes on each side, then place on a plate to rest for 5 minutes while cooking the veg.
3. Heat the remaining sesame oil in a wok over a high heat. Add the onion, red pepper and Chinese cabbage and stir-fry for 2 minutes. Add the shiitake and stir-fry for a further 2 minutes. Turn off the heat and add the steak.

Serve topped with the cashew nuts.

VARIATIONS: If you have it, you can use ketjap manis, a thick and syrupy spiced soy sauce used in Indonesian cooking. You can also replace the steak with cubed tofu for an equally fragrant vegetarian version with a lower calorie count.

PLENTY DAY SUGGESTION: Add a 40g serving of wholegrain basmati rice (40g uncooked weight), which will give a total of 484 calories and a new protein content of 30.4g.

Speedy Chicken Tikka Masala

320 calories, 37g protein, 4 portions of veg

This recipe is fast and also very adaptable. The same method can be used for other flavours – chipotle paste makes a smoky chicken dish with a Latin American flavour, while hot harissa paste is Moroccan style (you don't need to use the yogurt for these but could add a handful of cooked black beans or chickpeas for even more diversity!).

Serves 2
Preparation time: 10 minutes plus marinating time (1 hour)
Cooking time: 12–13 minutes

240g chicken breast fillets
10ml coconut oil or other cooking oil
1 small red onion, chopped
1 red pepper, chopped
200g cherry tomatoes, roughly chopped
200g cauliflower, broken into small florets
75ml Greek-style yogurt or coconut yogurt
For the tikka paste (or use 3 tbsp ready-made tikka paste):
1 tsp coriander seeds
2 garlic cloves
1 tsp turmeric
1 tsp cayenne pepper
1 chilli pepper
2 tbsp double-concentrate tomato purée

To serve:
Fresh coriander, to garnish

1. For home-made tikka paste: place all the paste ingredients in the container of a stick blender (or a tall jug: you don't want chilli or garlic in your eye). Blend together until the whole mix is thick and fragrant.
2. Cut the chicken into bite-sized pieces and then mix it into half of the ready-made or home-made paste to coat. Let it marinate in the fridge for 1 hour, or overnight if you have time (the easiest way is to use a plastic box or sealable bag).
3. Fry the marinated chicken pieces in half the oil till cooked through, around 5–7 minutes. Now add the rest of the oil and the vegetables and cook for another 2 minutes.
4. Add the rest of the paste, plus 100ml water. Cook, stirring gently, for 4–5 minutes until the cauliflower is just tender and the tomatoes break down and create a thicker sauce.
5. Stir the yogurt through just before serving and sprinkle over the coriander as a garnish.

VARIATIONS: For a veggie or vegan version, make with 200g cubed paneer or tofu. The Apetina variety of paneer is tasty but lower in fat than some paneer, or use firm, unsmoked tofu. The paneer version is 348 calories and 30g protein, and the tofu version will be around 290 calories with around 20g protein.

PLENTY DAY SUGGESTION: To serve 2, add 80g (dry weight) wholegrain basmati rice, cooked for 20–25 minutes, (adds 142 calories/3.6g protein per serving).

Barley Pot with Balsamic and Mustard Roast Winter Roots

354 calories, 11g protein, 5 portions veg

Pearl barley makes a base for a hearty, gut-friendly supper, a little like risotto. But it's easier as you don't have to keep stirring all the time! This has sweetness and heat from the mustard. It also reheats well the next day in the microwave if you need to use up the second portion.

Serves 2

Preparation time: 10 minutes

Cooking time: 35–40 minutes

80g uncooked pearl barley

500ml vegetable stock made with 2 tsp vegetable bouillon powder

1 large carrot

1 small parsnip or 2 baby parsnips (90g)

140g raw beetroot (2 small), peeled, tops cut off

1 red onion

7g butter/oil

2 portobello mushrooms

2 tbsp balsamic vinegar

2 tsp Dijon mustard

3 tbsp cooked, tinned pinto or red kidney beans, drained

To serve:

Fresh herbs

1. Preheat the oven to 220°C/200°C fan/425°F/Gas mark 7. Rinse the barley, add to a pan with the stock, bring to the boil then simmer for 30–35 minutes: top up with more water if needed.
2. Cut all the veg except the mushrooms into even-sized cubes/pieces around 2cm square. Scatter into a shallow baking dish. Dot the oil or butter over the veg, season, and roast for 15 minutes. Check and add a splash of water if the veg look very dry, and turn down the temperature to 200°C/180°C fan/400°F/Gas mark 6 if they're browning too much. Add mushrooms to the top and roast with the rest of the veg for another 15 minutes.
3. When the barley is cooked, add the pinto or kidney beans to the pan and warm through. Cut the cooked mushrooms into quarters and place on top of the barley and beans, with the rest of the roast veg. Whisk together the balsamic vinegar and mustard and pour over the dish. Garnish with fresh herbs and serve.

PLENTY DAY SUGGESTIONS: Just like risotto, this is a very versatile dish – try scattering over blue cheese or adding lean sausages or bacon to the roasting veg.

Hot Lamb Meatballs with Red Slaw and Cinna-Mint Drizzle

349 calories, 22g protein, 2 portions of veg

These little kofta-style meatballs are easy to make and the jalapeños give them a lovely kick. Add red slaw and a probiotic kefir drizzle and you've got a tasty, light meal you can share.

Serves 4
Preparation time: 10 minutes (plus 20 minutes chilling)
Cooking time: 10 minutes

For the meatballs:
350g 20% fat lamb mince
2 garlic cloves, crushed
1 tsp ground cayenne pepper
1 tsp ground cumin
1 medium egg, beaten
50g light cottage cheese, crumbled
20g sliced green jalapeños from a jar, drained and finely chopped
1 tsp oil
2 little gem lettuces or 1 romaine lettuce, leaves shredded

For the cinna-mint drizzle:
100ml kefir
¼ tsp ground cinnamon
5g fresh mint

For the slaw:

180g red cabbage, shredded

1 medium red onion, finely sliced

1 tsp extra-virgin olive oil

Juice of 1 lemon

200g raw peeled beetroot (or vacuum-packed), grated or finely sliced

To serve:

50g pomegranate seeds

1. For the meatballs, mix together the lamb mince, garlic, spices, egg, cheese and chopped jalapeños in a bowl and season well. Use a heaped teaspoon to form walnut-sized balls (around 4 per person) and place on an oiled baking sheet and put in the fridge to chill for 20 minutes.

2. Heat the grill to high and grill the lamb balls for 8–10 minutes, until golden brown and cooked through.

3. To make the slaw, combine all the ingredients. To make the cinna-mint drizzle, blend the kefir, cinnamon and mint in a hand blender, or chop the mint very finely and combine with the kefir and cinnamon in a bowl. Season to taste.

4. To serve, arrange the lettuce and the slaw on a plate. Place the meatballs on top, drizzle over the kefir sauce and top with the pomegranate seeds.

To use frozen mince: cook the frozen mince in a frying pan without fat for 10 minutes (or as per pack instructions) with the spices and garlic. Allow to cool slightly in the pan. Transfer to a bowl with the crumbled cheese and beaten egg, mix together and season. Use a heaped teaspoon to form the mix into 16 balls (4 per serving). Add 1 teaspoon of oil to the pan and fry for 2 minutes on each side.

PLENTY DAY SUGGESTIONS: Warmed mini wholemeal pittas are a nice addition (61 calories each, with 2.4g protein).

Mushroom and Black Bean Koftas with Cinna-Mint Drizzle, Red Slaw and Pitta Breads

268 calories, 13.4g protein, 3 portions of veg

These are really filling and tasty – they're soft inside, with little crumbs of cheese, and the low calorie count means you can serve with lots of extras.

Serves 4

Preparation time: 10 minutes (plus 10 minutes chilling)

Cooking time: 12–15 minutes

20g dried shiitake mushrooms

2 tsp extra-virgin olive oil

250g chestnut mushrooms, finely chopped

1 medium red onion, chopped

1 tsp cumin

1 tsp cayenne pepper

1 x 400g can black beans in water, drained

50g light feta cheese (or use tofu for a vegan/dairy-free version)

30g breadcrumbs

20g sliced green jalapeños from a jar, drained, finely chopped

For the cinna-mint drizzle:

100ml dairy or coconut kefir

10g fresh mint
¼ tsp ground cinnamon

For the slaw:
180g red cabbage, shredded
1 medium red onion, finely sliced
1 tsp extra-virgin olive oil
Juice of 1 lemon
200g raw peeled beetroot (or vacuum packed), grated or
finely sliced

To serve:
50g pomegranate seeds
4 wholemeal mini pitta breads

1. Soak the shiitake mushrooms in 75ml hot water for at least
   10 minutes while you prepare the other vegetables. Fry the
   fresh mushrooms, onion and spices in 1 teaspoon olive oil
   till lightly browned, around 5 minutes – add the shiitakes
   and soaking liquid at the end of cooking and allow liquid to
   evaporate.
2. Lightly mash the black beans with a fork and add the
   cheese, hot mushroom and onion mix, breadcrumbs and
   jalapeños.
3. Let the mix chill in the fridge for 10 minutes while you
   make the slaw. Place the koftas on a baking sheet, brush
   with oil using a pastry brush and grill for 8–10 minutes,
   turning halfway through, till koftas are golden brown and
   cooked through. At the end of cooking, sprinkle mini pittas

with a little water and grill till they just puff up.

4. To make the slaw, combine all the ingredients. To make the cinna-mint drizzle, blend the kefir, cinnamon and mint in a hand blender, or chop the mint very finely and combine with the kefir and cinnamon in a bowl. Season to taste.

5. To serve, arrange the lettuce and the slaw on a plate. Open one pitta per plate and arrange the koftas to the side. Drizzle over the kefir sauce and top with the pomegranate seeds.

VARIATIONS: You can use any kind of bean with the mix and vary the spicing – or try smoked cheese instead of the feta. You can also fry the koftas lightly, 4 minutes each side, in the olive oil, for a slightly crispier texture.

Warm Puy Lentil Salad with Jewel Veg and Chilli Dressing

317 calories, 20g protein, 2.5 portions of veg

Pouches of pulses and grains are a godsend when you're short of time, so you can make a high-fibre, tasty meal with minimal fuss. This recipe came to be on a night I didn't fancy a stir fry, so I used a stir-fry mix with lentils and an aromatic dressing. NB: It's made for 2 because that works best with a ready-cooked pouch, and the second helping can be kept in the fridge.

Serves 2
Preparation time: 5 minutes
Cooking time: 3 minutes

1 pack broccoli, baby corn and sugar snap stir-fry veg (240g)
1 250g pack pre-cooked Puy lentils
1 tsp sesame oil
1 tbsp rice wine vinegar or soy sauce
1 garlic clove, crushed
1 small red chilli, deseeded, finely chopped, or a good pinch dried chilli flakes
80g smoked tofu, cut into small cubes OR 1 hard-boiled egg, finely chopped

To serve:
Green tops of spring onions or fresh basil to garnish

1. Bring a large pan of water to the boil. Cook the stir-fry veg for around 3 minutes till just tender.
2. Meanwhile, microwave the lentils according to the packet instructions. Make the dressing by combining the oil, vinegar or soy, garlic and chilli.
3. Drain the vegetables and place in a bowl with the cooked lentils. Mix together, pour over the dressing. Season and sprinkle over the tofu or egg (if you like, you can dry-fry the tofu till browned).

VARIATION: If you'd rather use dried lentils, use 100g. Rinse them and place with a bay leaf in a saucepan, covered with 200ml water. Bring to the boil, then reduce to a simmer and cook for 20–25 minutes until the lentils are cooked but still have 'bite'. Top up water levels as the lentils cook so they don't burn.

PLENTY DAY SUGGESTIONS: Serve with a grilled or oven-baked chicken breast or cod fillet.

Smoked Salmon Spaghetti and Courgette with Creamy Watercress Sauce

392 calories, 24g protein, 2 portions of veg

A really luxurious and generous treat for one – or double up to serve a friend too. The courgette is uncooked to give a good crunch to the dish – I use a small julienne peeler rather than a cumbersome spiraliser.

Serves 1

Preparation time: 10 minutes

Cooking time: 10 minutes

65g wholewheat or spelt spaghetti

5g pine nuts

50g watercress or baby spinach

50ml full-fat Greek yogurt

1 small courgette, cut into julienne strips or spiralised

40g smoked salmon pieces

1. Cook the spaghetti in a large pan of boiling salted water according to the packet instructions. Drain (reserving a cupful of the cooking water) and set aside.
2. While the pasta is cooking, gently toast the pine nuts under the grill or in a dry pan – watch closely as they are quick to burn.
3. Place two-thirds of the watercress and the yogurt in a cup or mug and use a hand blender to create a smooth

sauce. Season with salt and pepper.

4. Stir the watercress sauce through the cooked linguini, adding a little of the reserved cooking water, as needed, to loosen the sauce. Gently mix in the reserved watercress, the courgette and the smoked salmon pieces and scatter the pine nuts on top. Serve in a warmed bowl.

VARIATION: For a vegetarian version, replace the smoked salmon with 20g sun-dried tomatoes or 30g artichoke hearts, cut into small pieces, and add 10g grated Grana Padano or veggie Italian-style cheese just before serving. Comes to 394 calories, 18g protein.

Fast Flatbread Pizza

Making a pizza base isn't hard but on a Fast Day you probably want something super quick. Use small folded flatbreads for this – it's the topping that matters; or if you use a slightly larger tortilla, just add in the extra calories. Do feel free to use any of your own toppings – these two are just a guide.

Hot Devil

325 calories, 14.3g protein, 2.5 portions of veg

1 seeded, folded flatbread or smaller tortilla (around 40g)

1 tbsp tomato puree

2 medium whole tomatoes (around 120g)

1 small red onion, sliced

10g jalapeño peppers from a jar, drained and chopped

100g roasted red peppers from a jar, drained and chopped

13g/3 slices pepperoni sausage, chopped or veggie equivalent

50g light mozzarella, torn or sliced into thin pieces

½ tsp extra-virgin olive oil

To serve:
Small handful fresh basil

Middle Eastern Veg

322 calories, 17g protein, 4 portions of veg

1 seeded, folded flatbread or smaller tortilla (around 40g)

2 tbsp double-concentrate tomato purée

1 large tomato (85g), sliced

1 small red onion, sliced

40g light cottage cheese, crumbled, or cubed tofu

4 stalks of tenderstem broccoli, steamed or boiled till just cooked

40g cooked broad beans

1 tsp extra-virgin olive oil

To serve:

10g pomegranate seeds

Small handful fresh mint

1. Preheat the oven to 200°C/ 220°C fan/400°F/gas mark 6. Preheat a baking tray in the oven for 5 minutes.
2. Unfold the wrap and place with folded side down on the tray (so it doesn't fold over again). Arrange all ingredients on top except fresh herbs (and pomegranate seeds for the Middle Eastern Veg) and drizzle over the olive oil.
3. Bake for 8–10 minutes directly on the oven shelf, with the tray underneath to catch any drips! Check to make sure ingredients don't burn and for a crisper topping, finish under a hot grill for 1 minute. Remove from oven, sprinkle over the fresh herbs, and pomegranate seeds if using, and serve immediately.

Main Dishes +

The next few dishes are a little higher in calories, but can work brilliantly if you're one of the many people who prefer to eat most of their allowance in single meal with friends and family. These calorie counts still allow you to enjoy a soup or side dish/salad as a smaller meal – and the dishes themselves are still wholesome and delicious, so they're perfect for your Plenty Days.

Bacon, Bean and Spinach Risotto with White Wine

475 calories, 17.4g protein, 2 portions of veg

Risotto is so comforting and this one tastes autumnal and earthy, with the beans and bacon. For a veggie version, use 2–3 veggie or Quorn sausages. See below for two variations, but once you've worked out the technique, you can add whatever you fancy. You can keep portions in the fridge to reheat – add the cheese just before serving.

Serves 4

Preparation time: 5 minutes

Cooking time: 22–30 minutes

2 tsp olive oil or butter

2 small onions, finely chopped

75g fennel or celery

4 thin rashers of lean back bacon, cut into bite-sized pieces

2 garlic cloves, finely chopped

300g Arborio risotto rice

120ml white wine

1 x 400g can cannellini or borlotti beans, drained

700ml hot chicken or vegetable stock (fresh, or from bouillon/stock cubes)

160g baby spinach

To serve:

25g grated Parmesan or Grana Padano, or veggie Italian cheese

1. Heat the oil or butter in a large saucepan and fry the onion, fennel or celery and bacon for 2–3 minutes over a medium heat, until softened but not coloured. Turn down the heat, add the garlic and fry for another minute.
2. Add the rice and stir through for 2 minutes. Turn up the heat, pour in the wine and cook for 1 minute, then begin adding the hot stock, a ladleful at a time, waiting until each one is absorbed before adding the next: the rice grains will gradually change colour and become opaque. Check the grains after about 14 minutes cooking time – they should be soft but not mushy. Add the beans towards the end of the cooking time, so they warm through but don't disintegrate.
3. When the rice is cooked, add the baby spinach and let it wilt.

VARIATIONS:

PRIMAVERA (VEGETARIAN OPTION): Instead of the bacon and fennel, use 300g asparagus, sliced into bite-sized chunks, 200g frozen peas and 100g frozen baby broad beans instead of the borlotti beans. Add 10g toasted pine nuts, and grate over a little lemon zest just before serving (464 calories per serving, 9.5g protein, 2.5 portions of veg).

PORCINI MUSHROOM AND LEEK (VEGETARIAN OPTION): Use 100g dried wild or shiitake mushrooms and 200g chopped chestnut mushrooms in place of the bacon, plus

2 medium leeks in place of the onion and fennel. Fry fresh mushrooms and leeks before adding the rice. Rehydrate 10g dried wild or porcini mushrooms in 100ml hot water, and add the soaked mushrooms and water to the risotto when you add the wine (387 calories per serving, 11g protein, 1.5 portions of veg).

Sticky Ginger Chicken/ Tofu with Turmeric Rice Noodles

473 calories. Chicken version: 50g protein; tofu version 18g protein.

Both 3 portions of veg

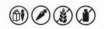

Delicious and easy – the rice noodles don't need cooking, just covering with boiling water and a little turmeric to turn them a lovely golden colour. If you remember to marinate the chicken or tofu in the fridge overnight, it'll taste even better. If you want to cut the calories down see Variations, below.

Serves 1

Preparation time: 10 minutes (plus 10 minutes/overnight to marinate)

Cooking time: 8 minutes

1 tsp sesame oil

1 tsp honey

1 tbsp soy sauce

1cm piece fresh ginger, grated

1 x 165g skinless chicken breast, or 150g tofu, cut into bite-sized chunks

3 spring onions, bulbs only, chopped or snipped into rounds

½ tsp ground turmeric

40g instant rice noodles

80g sugar snap peas

4 stalks Tenderstem broccoli, cut into bite-sized pieces

60g green beans or French beans

To serve (optional):

1 tsp sesame seeds

1 small red chilli cut into rings, to garnish

1. Mix together the oil, honey, soy sauce and ginger in a lidded plastic food container. Add the chicken or tofu, replace the lid and shake to cover. Let it marinate in the fridge, overnight or for at least 10 minutes.
2. When you're ready to eat, heat a large non-stick frying pan and tip the chicken/tofu and marinade into the pan. Add the spring onion, and cook until the chicken browns and is almost cooked through, around 5 minutes depending on the size of the pieces. It'll take less time for the tofu, which tastes best browned at the edges.
3. Meanwhile, place the noodles in a small bowl and boil the kettle. Pour in enough boiling water to cover and stir in the turmeric. Most instant noodles take 3–4 minutes to be ready.
4. Add the other vegetables to the pan with around 100ml water. Turn up the heat, cover the pan, and let the vegetables steam for about a minute. Remove the lid to let any water evaporate, then add the noodles to the pan and mix well till warmed through.
5. Serve with sesame seeds and/or chilli sprinkled over the top.

VARIATIONS: On a Fast Day, cut back on the chicken or tofu to 100g uncooked, and reduce the rice noodle portion to 20g: the calorie count comes down to 355, with 34g protein for the chicken version, 21g for the tofu dish.

Chicken Pasta Bake with Ricotta, Lemon and Veggies

477 calories, 43g protein, 3 portions of veg

This is easy, filling and makes a creamy and zingy change from the usual tomato-based pasta bakes: it was a real favourite among our test dieters. You can also bake in individual baking tins or dishes.

Serves 4
Preparation time: 10 minutes
Cooking time: 30 minutes

140g wholewheat pasta shapes, e.g. penne

400g skinless chicken breast fillets

300g raw butternut squash

1 red onion, chopped

250g chestnut mushrooms, sliced

1 tsp olive oil or butter

3 garlic cloves

240g young spinach leaves

400g ricotta

Zest of 1 lemon

60ml kefir or whole milk

30g Grana Padano or Parmesan cheese

1. Preheat the oven to 200°C/220°C fan/400°F/gas mark 6. Cook pasta for 5 minutes and drain to stop further cooking.

2. Chop the chicken and the squash into bite-sized pieces. Fry the onion, mushrooms and squash in the oil or butter in a large pan for 2 minutes, then add the chicken pieces and garlic and cook for 6 minutes: add a splash of water if it's a little dry. Add the spinach leaves and cook for a minute or so till they wilt in the pan. Take off the heat.
3. Whip together half the ricotta with the lemon zest and kefir or milk. Add to the pan and mix well.
4. Pile the pasta mix into a baking dish and top with the remaining ricotta, making sure to spread it well so it covers most of the pasta to prevent it burning. Grate over the hard cheese and bake for 15 minutes.

VARIATIONS: If you want to serve on a Fast Day, divide into 6 portions – it comes down to 318 calories, ideal served with a good bunch of rocket leaves dressed with balsamic vinegar.

For a tomato and ricotta version, at step 3 mix the chicken and vegetables with 1 can of chopped Italian tomatoes and use *all* the ricotta mix as a topping. This adds around 20 calories per serving for 4 people.

Side dishes and sweet things

In this section I've included fantastic side dishes which make a meal even more satisfying – plus a handful of sweet ends to a meal that are quick to prepare and taste yummy.

Refried Beans with White Cheese and Coriander

107 calories, 6.4g protein, 1 portion of veg

'Refried' beans aren't really refried, and don't even have to be fried at all. Just beans, lightly mashed and warmed with onion, garlic and spices. In Mexico, they often use pinto beans, but black beans are higher in phytonutrients, and I love the contrast with the white cheese. They're a lovely accompaniment to anything with Mexican flavours or as a topping for a jacket potato, a dip or light lunch with some Little Gem lettuce leaves.

Makes 4 portions (store in the fridge)
Preparation time: 5 minutes
Cooking time: 6 minutes

1 small onion, finely chopped

1 tsp ground cumin

1 tsp butter or olive oil (or, to be authentic, lard)

2 garlic cloves, crushed

1 x 400g can pinto or black beans, drained

½–1 tsp chilli or cayenne powder (optional)

To serve:
30g crumbled Lancashire or feta cheese, for topping
Optional: Fresh coriander

1. Fry the onion with the cumin in the butter or oil for 4–5 minutes till translucent. Add the garlic and fry for another minute, then stir in the drained beans to warm through.
2. Roughly mash the beans with a fork in the pan – or if you want a smoother dip consistency, use a hand blender. Season and add chilli or cayenne if using.
3. Divide up the crumbled cheese and scatter over each portion, with the fresh coriander leaves if using. Serve cool or warm as a dip or sandwich filling or with crudités or Little Gem leaves. Also great as a side with any Mexican dish.

VARIATIONS: use fresh chilli – fry with the onion – and top with 30g coconut yogurt for a vegan version with a kick.

Crunchy Sweet Slaw with Dill and Caraway

88 calories, 3g protein, 2 portions of veg

Everywhere you look on trendy menus, there's 'slaw' – and it's a long way from the family-sized tubs of cabbage and carrot in gloopy, over-sweet mayo. Slaw is basically a salad of chopped vegetables in a dressing: it often contains cabbage, but that's not compulsory. Your home-made versions can be anything you want. But this is a tangy, crunchy start; prebiotic and probiotic, thanks to the kefir and the cabbage.

Makes 4 portions
Preparation time: 10 minutes

250g shredded white or red cabbage
2 medium carrots, grated or finely sliced
1 small apple and 1 small pear (or 2 of either), grated or finely sliced
10ml cider vinegar
100ml kefir
1 tsp caraway seeds
To serve:
1 tsp chopped fresh dill or parsley
15g pumpkin seeds

1. Combine the vegetables in a bowl. Mix the vinegar, kefir and caraway seeds together, then pour over the vegetables and stir through.

2. Top with the fresh herbs and pumpkin seeds.

**VARIATIONS: You can also mix in some fermented cabbage
(e.g. the home-made sauerkraut on p. 295 with fresh
cabbage) for a tangier, delicious variation.**

Kale Salad with Peas and Pesto Flavour

129 calories, 8.1g protein, 1.5 portions of veg

This tasty salad is filling and delicious, thanks to the strong flavours and high protein count. Massaging helps to slightly soften the kale, making it easier to eat!

Serves 2

Preparation time: 10 minutes

125g cavolo nero or kale, washed, tough stems removed

1 tsp olive oil

¼ tsp sea salt and pepper

Juice and rind of 1 lemon

100g cooked peas

Good handful fresh basil

To serve:

10g Parmesan or Grana Padano, or veggie Italian cheese, grated

7g pine nuts, toasted in a dry pan or under grill

1. Place the kale leaves in a bowl with the olive oil, salt and lemon juice. With clean hands, massage the dressing into the leaves, until they begin to soften up and are well coated. Tear into bite-sized pieces
2. Mix in the peas and basil leaves, season with pepper and sprinkle over grated cheese and pine nuts before serving.

VARIATIONS: Try the same dish with lime juice and sesame oil, plus cubes of smoked tofu and crushed peanuts; or orange juice and rind, cubed blue cheese, olive oil and poppy seeds.

Purple Sprouting Broccoli with Romesco Sauce

154 calories, 6.8g protein, 2.5 portions of veg

(leave out sourdough bread)

I love spicy, sharp, nutty Romesco sauce, and it goes so well with grilled or lightly charred vegetables like broccoli – the purple sprouting kind looks amazing on the plate. But you can serve this with any vegetable, or the sauce is also delicious with grilled fish or chicken, or cooked, cooled salad potatoes.

Serves 4

Preparation time: 12 minutes

Cooking time: 20 minutes

400g purple sprouting broccoli

For the sauce:

100g tomatoes

2 garlic cloves, unpeeled

1 small red or green chilli pepper

1 red pepper, halved

40g day-old country-style or sourdough bread

2 tbsp sherry vinegar or red wine vinegar

1 tsp smoked paprika

20g almonds or hazelnuts

Small handful fresh parsley

1 tbsp extra-virgin olive oil

1. For the sauce, preheat the grill to high. Line a grill pan with foil and add the tomatoes, garlic, chilli and pepper halves. Grill for around 10 minutes, turning the veg over halfway through. Add the bread to the grill pan in the last couple of minutes so it browns but does not burn.

2. Place the grilled vegetables in a bowl. When cool enough to handle, slip off the garlic, tomato and pepper skins and break open the pepper and chilli with your fingers to remove the cores and seeds (wash your hands afterwards!).

3. In a food processor, blend the bread to crumbs, then add the vegetables, but only half the chilli pepper, the vinegar and the paprika. Process to a paste and set aside.

4. Toast the nuts in a dry non-stick pan till they brown then add those to the processor and pulse until roughly ground. Finally add the parsley and 10ml of the olive oil and process till it makes a sauce/paste. Taste and add the second half of the chilli pepper if you like a hotter sauce.

5. Blanch the broccoli in boiling water for 3 minutes. Cut in half lengthwise. Apply a little oil, griddle or fry till softened, and charring slightly around the edges: around 5–7 minutes. Season with sea salt and black pepper.

6. Serve the veg with the sauce poured over or as a dip.

VARIATION: Try making with different nuts e.g. walnuts or pecans. You can make this more speedily by using chipotle paste, fresh garlic and roasted red peppers from a jar – wipe the peppers with kitchen roll to take away excess oil.

Sweet Potato, Lime and Turmeric Wedges

139 calories, 1.8g protein, 1 portion of veg

Exactly as they sound – a lovely side or starter (try serving with the tzatziki from p. 195). Good for making for a crowd or when you're roasting something else. If you ever see purple sweet potatoes, they're even more rich in antioxidants.

Serves 2

Preparation time: 5 minutes

Cooking time: 30–35 minutes

2 small sweet potatoes (around 125g each)

Juice of ½ a lime

1 tsp turmeric

1 tsp oil, e.g. sesame, rapeseed, coconut

1. Pre-heat the oven to 200°C/220°C fan/400°F/Gas mark 6. Scrub but don't peel the sweet potatoes. Cut into small wedges – each potato makes about 12–16.
2. Squeeze the juice into a large baking dish, add the turmeric and oil (if it's coconut oil, you'll need to warm it in the oven as it's solid at room temperature). Place the wedges in the tray, turn to coat in the juice and oil, and roast for 30–35 minutes, turning once.

VARIATIONS: For a cauliflower version, use 300g cauliflower florets – steam or boil them till just tender. Coat in the oil and lime mix as for the potatoes, but roast for around 20 minutes, till they're dark brown but not burned at the edges (this version is 87 calories per serving).

Summer Berries with Kefir Cheesecake Topping

142 calories, 4.3g protein, 2 portions of fruit

(with oat biscuits)

I love cheesecake but a wedge of it can be really heavy and pretty high in calories. This puts ripe summer fruit centre-stage, but gives a cheesecake flavour, with almonds, biscuit crumbs and sweet-sour kefir.

Serves 2
Preparation time: 5 minutes

150g strawberries
150g raspberries
¼ tsp vanilla extract
60ml dairy or coconut kefir
10g flaked or whole almonds
2 wholemeal digestive or oat biscuits

1. Cut the strawberries into bite-sized pieces and place in two serving bowls with the raspberries. Mix the vanilla extract with the kefir.
2. Toast the almonds in a dry pan – watch them so they don't burn. Crush them with the biscuits.
3. Pour the kefir over the fruit and then sprinkle over the nut-and-biscuit mix.

VARIATION: Use tropical fruit like mango, pineapple or passion fruit, with crushed pecans and ginger biscuits.

Little Kefir Parfait Shot

62 calories, 2.7g protein

Dessert Black Berries Parfait Pot

155 calories, 5.7g protein, 2 portions of fruit

This is a great way to create a sweet dessert or treat that is just brilliant for your gut. There are two options: chia seeds (much loved by clean eaters but that shouldn't put you off!) or oats. There are two versions here – one works well as a Fast Day bio extra. The other is more substantial.

Serves 1
Preparation time: 3 minutes plus chilling time (1 hour-overnight)

For the Little Kefir Parfait Shot:
60ml kefir
4g chia seeds OR 5g rolled oats
30g blueberries or other berries

For the Dessert Black Berries Kefir Parfait Pot:
100ml kefir
4g chia seeds OR 5g rolled oats
50g blueberries
50g blackberries
50g blackcurrants
1 tsp honey, agave or maple syrup
3 pistachio nuts, lightly crushed

1. Pour the kefir over the chia or oats and mix through the honey/syrup if using. Chill in the fridge for at least an hour, or overnight.
2. Mix through the fruit and top with nuts if using.

VARIATIONS: Try with any of the combinations listed in the Heart-Warmer Porridge or Overnight Power Oats recipes in the Breakfast and Brunches section (p. 149).

Dark Chocolate Ginger and Apricot Truffles

27 calories, 0.6g protein per truffle

These are wonderfully bittersweet, because they use the darkest chocolate, with sweetness from dried fruit, and a hint of spice. I roll these and place in little petit four cases and store them in the freezer so I only take out one at a time . . .

Makes 18 truffles

Preparation time: 15 minutes, plus soaking and chilling time

Cooking time: 5 minutes (or 2 minutes in the microwave)

25g dried apricots

25g walnuts

50g dark chocolate (90% cocoa solids), broken into pieces

½–1 tsp ground ginger

1 tsp unsweetened cocoa powder (optional)

1. Put the apricots into a small dish and cover with 25ml boiling water. Set aside to soak for 30 minutes.
2. Whiz the walnuts in a small food processor until finely ground, then tip into a bowl. Process the apricots with any leftover water into a purée.
3. Melt the chocolate in a small bowl resting over a saucepan of boiling water (make sure the base of the bowl doesn't

touch the water). If you have a microwave it's easier: heat for 30 seconds at a time in a microwaveable container until melted.

4. Stir in the nuts, the ginger and then the purée, till well mixed. Cover and chill in the fridge for 4 hours or overnight.

5. The next day, wash your hands, then scoop up about 1 scant teaspoon of the mixture at a time and roll it into a ball in your hands. If you want, sprinkle unsweetened cocoa powder on a plate or work surface and roll the balls in that before placing on a plate or into petit four cases. Your hands will be messy (don't do this on a Fast Day – the temptation may be too much!) but the chocolate will melt on contact enough to create neat balls.

6. Repeat until you've made 18 balls. Store in a re-sealable container in the fridge for up to a week or freeze for up to 3 months.

VARIATIONS: Swap the nuts, dried fruit and spices: try chilli and pineapple or cinnamon and cranberry (try to use dried fruits with no added sugars). You can also use ground seed mixes e.g. flaxseed and walnut.

Quick calorie counter and ideas for Dirty Diet-friendly foods

●

This counter gives the calorie counts and suggested portion sizes for a range of different foods, plus lots of serving ideas and suggestions for additions which turn two or three ingredients into something really special.

Note: whether a food is prebiotic or not varies depending on the quantity and type of fibre. We've highlighted the best ones as 'Prebiotic' in the relevant column, while foods which have prebiotic potential if eaten in large portions or in combination with others are listed as 'Can be prebiotic'. N.B. most grains and starches can be prebiotic due to resistant starch if cooked then allowed to cool e.g. potatoes and rice used in salad, cooked pasta used in salad or in dishes where it has been cooked, cooled and reheated; and many varieties of cheese can be probiotic if made with unpasteurised milk, or made using natural methods (e.g. some farmhouse cheeses), aged, or with visible moulds like blue cheese.

What	Size	Calories	Serving ideas	Probiotic/ prebiotic?
Vegetables				
Artichoke hearts	½ 390g can, drained	36	Grilled with blue cheese	Prebiotic
Artichokes (Jerusalem)	100g	41	Boiled or roasted with a little olive oil	Prebiotic
Asparagus	100g	27	With a poached egg	Prebiotic
Avocado	medium, half	135–145	With balsamic vinegar or lemon juice	
Raw or steamed cauliflower	100g, 4–5 florets	25	With chilli sauce With grated cheese Pan-grilled with whole spices, e.g. mustard seeds	
Raw or steamed broccoli	85g	29	With soy or tamari With romesco sauce	
Beans, French or fine green	100g	30	With toasted almonds	
Beetroot	125g (half a vacuum pack in water)	52	With chilli dressing and orange	
Courgette	1 medium (170g)	34	As courgetti/noodles with lemon zest, chillies and 1 tsp olive oil	
Cucumber	100g	14	With chilli, salt, wasabi sauce	Can be prebiotic
Edamame beans	50g	65	With fresh pepper, soy sauce, chilli sauce	
Fennel	80g	10	Finely sliced with lemon juice and olive oil as a side dish	Prebiotic

What	Size	Calories	Serving ideas	Probiotic/ prebiotic?
Little Gem or romaine lettuce	1 small Little Gem	15	Used as a wrap for dips and sandwich fillings	
Mushrooms, portobello	1 medium	18	Grilled with pizza herbs, and 1 tsp olive oil	Can be prebiotic
Mushrooms, shiitake	100g	35–40	Fried or grilled with 1 tsp sesame oil	Can be prebiotic
Onions	1 small	38–50	Pickle red onions in fresh lime juice	Prebiotic
Spring onions	1 small	2	Grilled with black pepper or Romesco sauce	Prebiotic
Rocket	25g	6	Dressed with balsamic or wine vinegar	
Seaweed, dressed	Dried 5g (rehydrates to 50g)	50	With sesame seeds or oil	Prebiotic
Seaweed crackers/ snacks	5g pack	20–25	Delicious on their own or with hummus	Prebiotic
Baby spinach	50g	8	With blue cheese or seeds	
Cooked frozen spinach	90g	19	Swirl of kefir/yogurt and spices/nutmeg	
Peas	80g	64	Lightly mashed with fresh mint	
Sugar snaps/ mangetout	80g	28–32	Stir-fried till just browning, in sesame or coconut oil, with a little soy sauce	
White potato	100g boiled 1 medium baked 180g	70–90 175	Top with blue cheese, slaw, black or baked beans	Prebiotic when cooked and cooled

What	Size	Calories	Serving ideas	Probiotic/ prebiotic?
Radish	8 radishes	8	With celery salt or horseradish	
Tomatoes	100g cherry medium	20 3–5 15–20	With a sprinkle of salt and pepper, plus 1 tsp olive oil and 1 tsp vinegar With finely chopped shallots	
Roasted or grilled tomatoes	100g	15–20	With balsamic vinegar With feta cheese	
Roast mixed vegetables	100g aubergine, peppers, courgette	25	With miso With balsamic vinegar	
Sweet potato	1 medium (175g)	152	Delicious with yogurt, cheese or garlic mushrooms	
Grains and bread				
Sourdough bread	1 x 50g slice	110–115		
Sourdough bread	1 thin 25g slice	55–58		
Wholegrain basmati rice	45g uncooked	160	Add beans to make rice and beans	Prebiotic after cooking and cooling
Wholegrain/ spelt pasta (small portion)	45g uncooked	155		Prebiotic when precooked and cooled
Freekeh (¼ pack)	60g	108		
Quinoa	½ 250g vacuum pack	235		
Poppadoms	1 cooked in microwave	35		

What	Size	Calories	Serving ideas	Probiotic/ prebiotic?
Oatcakes	1	45–50		Prebiotic
Cream crackers	1	35		
Popcorn	15g uncooked	46		
Pulses				
Puy lentils (¼ pack)	60g	86		Prebiotic
Canned chickpeas, black beans, lentils	¼ 400g can, drained	60–80		Prebiotic
Baked beans (Heinz)	100g	79		Prebiotic
Nuts (all raw, unsalted)				
Almonds	17 or 18	100		
Brazil nuts	5 medium	100		
Cashews	13 or 14	100		
Peanuts	30 small	100		
Pistachios	25–28	100		
Pecans	10	100		
Walnuts	6	100		
Pumpkin seeds	1 tsp	29		
Sunflower seeds	1 tsp	32		
Other				
Olives, pitted black in brine, drained	10	38	Marinate in orange juice and zest, or garlic and a little oil (garlic is prebiotic)	Prebiotic

What	Size	Calories	Serving ideas	Probiotic/ prebiotic?
Fruits				
Apple	1	50–70		Can be prebiotic
Apricot, fresh	1	17		Can be prebiotic
Orange or blood orange	1 medium	58–70	Serve in a savoury salad with beetroot and red onion	
Banana	1 medium	100	With peanut butter and dates With Greek yogurt	Prebiotic
Blueberries	50g	29	Great in sweet and savoury dishes	
Cherries	10	50		Can be prebiotic
Dates	1 small (7g without stone)	19		Can be prebiotic
Grapefruit	1 medium	60	With avocado as a salad	
Grapes	10	34		
Mini or golden kiwis	1	42		
Passion fruit	1	17	As a sauce over other fruit	
Peach/ nectarine	1 medium	51		
Pear	1 small (120g)	48		Can be prebiotic
Pineapple	30g slice	14		
Pomegranate seeds	15g	15		

What	Size	Calories	Serving ideas	Probiotic/ prebiotic?
Rhubarb	50g stewed (no sugar)	4		
Blackberries	50g	20		Can be prebiotic
Strawberries	50g	16	With black pepper or balsamic vinegar	
Raspberries	50g	26		
Tangerine/ clementine	1	40		
Mango	½ medium mango (100–150g fruit)	60–90	With lime juice With banana With passion fruit	Can be prebiotic
Dairy and alternatives				
Greek yogurt	100ml	130		Probiotic
Coconut yogurt	100ml	55–195		Can be probiotic
Milk kefir	75ml	44		Probiotic
Coconut kefir	75ml	26		Probiotic
Cheddar, Lancashire, Leicester – hard cheese Reduced-fat blue cheese	25g (small matchbox-size piece)	93–110 70–80		Blue and aged unpasteurised cheese can be pro
Brie/ camembert Reduced fat	25g	75–85 55–60		Blue and aged unpasteurised cheese can be pro
Mozzarella Lower-fat	½ ball	170–180 100–110		Blue and aged unpasteurised cheese can be pro

What	Size	Calories	Serving ideas	Probiotic/prebiotic?
Halloumi Lower-fat		75–80 55		Blue and aged unpasteurised cheese can be pro
Feta Lower-fat		60–75 40–45		Can be probiotic
Proteins				
Ham	32g slice	44		
Chicken	100g raw breast meat	105		
Tuna	92g tinned	100		
Tofu	100g	115–125		
Jerky	20g (½ pack)	56–60		
Chicken pâté	40g	100–125		
Spreads and dips				
Tahini	10g	60		
Peanut butter	15g	90		
Hummus (shop-bought)	30g	90		Prebiotic
Reduced-fat hummus (shop-bought)	30g	70		Prebiotic
Tzatziki (shop-bought)	50g	60		Can be pro

Bliss Moments – these are examples only, as different brands can have very different calorie counts, especially with baked goods and savoury snacks. Do check your own favourites!

What	Size	Calories	What	Size	Calories
Small red wine	125ml	85	Individual lemon tart	1	300–400
Small glass dry cava, Prosecco, Champagne	125ml	95	Small slice chocolate cake	75g	315
Small dry white wine	125ml	85	Ice cream	2 standard soft scoops (86g) 2 luxury scoops (86g)	53 220–240
Spirit, single-measure, with 0-cal Slimline mixer	25ml for measure	56	Mini Magnum	1	160–175
Half-pint lager		80–122	Solero	1	95
Half-pint bitter		70–133	Cornetto	1	185
Half-pint dry cider		100–120	Scone	1	240–275
Normal mixer, e.g. tonic	150ml	33	Cupcake with icing	1 small (90g)	280–400
Fresh orange juice	125ml	45–55	Small pack crisps/ snacks from multipack	25g	120–145
Fresh apple juice	125ml	48–60	Pringles	40g (small pack)	200
Dark chocolate	25g	125–143			
Oat biscuit	1 small	50–60			
Chocolate digestive	1	83	Tortilla chips	40g pack	200
Muffin	1	300–450			

Probiotic foods: how to buy or make 'living' foods

Probiotic foods are alive – they help put back the good bacteria that modern processed diets, and antibiotics, may have removed. They're a kind of magic! In this section, we'll look at four kinds – what they are and why they're great:

- Yogurt
- Kefir
- Fermented vegetables
- Sourdough bread (which is not probiotic when baked but uses good bacteria to make the bread easier to digest)

They all involve a fermentation – converting the sugars in food into acid, alcohol or gases (the gases are why fermented food and drink is often slightly fizzy). It's bacteria and yeasts that do the fermenting – and by pre-digesting the food for us, they also make its nutrients more available to our bodies. These 'ferments' have been enjoyed for many centuries as the process helps to preserve fresh food. It's a win-win situation.

Making your own vs buying probiotic foods

While it's getting easier and easier to find good-quality probiotic foods, there are reasons to make your own:

- It's usually cheaper long term (though you may need to buy some simple kitchen items or starter cultures);
- It's satisfying to see how the foods come to life and understand how the good bacteria can work so well for us;
- It's much more customisable – you can choose the length of fermentation time and the intensity of flavour.

I see my little collection of live foods or ferments as tiny pets – I meet their basic needs and they give me so much in return. But if you remember the little Tamagotchi toys that were all the rage a few years ago, they're like those – pay them a little attention and they thrive. Ignore them and they die off, or go rogue! Fermenting can be hit-and-miss, and it also takes up space on kitchen worktops, so it's not compulsory by any means. If you don't fancy experimenting yourself, each section also offers hints on buying these great foods ready-made.

NB: Some people with lactose intolerance do find they can consume yogurt and kefir because the beneficial bacteria have digested most of the lactose. If you do want to try, start carefully with small quantities and listen to your body – if you have side-effects, stop eating. If you find live foods difficult to tolerate you can consider a probiotic supplement instead (see p. 320).

Yogurt

Yogurt is probably the most familiar of the probiotic foods we're talking about in this book: but I definitely don't mean over-sweetened or low-cal options. The yogurts we recommend are the plain, and usually full-fat, Greek versions.

Like cheese, yogurt is a great food to eat in small portions if you're watching your weight, as the balance of protein and fat means it makes you feel full and satisfied. But yogurt also contains microbes that are good for gut health.

Buying yogurt

Look at the labels next time you go shopping – some manufacturers have started to label the cultures or bacteria you'll find in the yogurts, which helps you to see that it's live. The most common tend to be from the lactobacillus group, and sometimes you'll also see Bifidobacterium and Streptococcus thermophilus listed.

Look for full-fat Greek or Greek-style (made in the same way, but not in Greece itself). Some flavoured yogurts are still full-fat and use only fruit as a sweetener, so those are an alternative. But watch out for high-calorie 'dessert' yogurts with added sugars or especially artificial sweeteners, which we don't recommend.

Making your own yogurt is a great straightforward introduction to the world of home fermentation. You'll be amazed how easy it is.

Making yogurt at home

Yogurt is really simple to make, and costs less than half the price of shop-bought, even if you use organic milk. You just need an insulated flask, milk and a little ready-made plain, live yogurt as a starter. I use Greek yogurt or re-use home-made.

For a thicker yogurt, use powdered milk – the sort you find in the supermarket by the UHT milks. The skimmed version is also fine to use. Without powdered milk, the yogurt will be runnier, but still taste delicious.

A cooking thermometer can help gauge temperatures, but personally I don't use one.

> 50ml/2 heaped tbsp live yogurt at room temperature to
> use as a starter
> 500ml fresh, full fat or semi-skimmed milk
> Optional: 1 heaped tablespoon of powdered milk

NB: wash all the equipment you're going to use in hot soapy water, especially the flask – you don't want the yogurt to smell of the tea you had yesterday!

1. Boil water in the kettle and pour into the flask or container to pre-heat it. Pour the milk into a pan and heat gently till the milk is starting to steam but doesn't boil. (If using a thermometer, the temperature to aim for is 85°C). This changes the structure of the milk molecules to allow them to make thicker yogurt.
2. Let the milk cool down till it's the temperature of a hot bath – not uncomfortable but definitely hot – test with a

clean finger. Or aim for a temperature of 46°C. Now whisk in the milk powder into the milk, if using, and then whisk in the yogurt.

3. Empty the hot water out of the flask. Pour the warm milk and yogurt mix into the flask. Replace the lid. Leave on the counter overnight or for at least eight hours. Check the texture and taste after that – the yogurt will thicken and become sourer the longer you leave it: I like it after about 18 hours. Once it's the taste and texture you prefer, decant into sterilised pots or jars and keep in the fridge for 5–7 days.

Remember to save a little of your home-made yogurt to make your next batch.

PS: if you don't have a flask, you can improvise with a heatproof container e.g. a Pyrex jar, and a blanket to keep the milk warm while the live starter gets to work. In step 3, pour the milk mix into your container, cover and then wrap up warm overnight or for 8+ hours!

Being able to include proper yogurt and cheese within my diet has been a revelation. I've always preferred normal, plain yogurt to overly sweetened fat-free ones. I was coming around to the idea that full-fat Greek or natural yogurt must be better for you than all those fake sweeteners, which always left a horrid taste in my mouth. Being on this plan has confirmed this for me and, honestly, I'd rather have a bowl of natural yogurt, fruit and a bit of honey or granola than chocolate.

Jenni

Kefir

Kefir is a fermented drink containing very high numbers of live bacteria, up to three times as many as in yogurt.

The main types are **water kefir** (which is made from sugar and water and makes a slightly fizzy drink), **coconut kefir** (made from fermenting coconut water or milk) and **dairy kefir**, which is a lot like drinking yogurt. In each case, the 'fizz' comes from the good bacteria acting on the sugars in the liquid – in the dairy and coconut versions, there's no added sugar.

We recommend **dairy or coconut kefir as the best all-round options**, but our bodies' responses will vary according to our existing gut bacteria. I actually had to stop drinking water kefir, even though I'd made delicious versions flavoured with ginger, lemon and berries. I really liked the flavour and the slight fizziness, but it gave me bad bloating. At times, it felt like I was going to go bang! I persevered for a few weeks, hoping my microbes would adjust, but it never happened. In contrast, I love dairy kefir and it loves me back.

It is a bit of a 'Marmite' ingredient that divided members of our first Dirty Diet panel. Many – including me – absolutely loved it, and found it was filling, versatile and had really positive effects on their gut health and digestion. But a small number didn't like it – finding the sour-ish yogurt smell and slight fizziness off-putting, and one reported that her digestion seemed worse after drinking it. Do consume smaller amounts of kefir for the first few days, to let your gut adjust to these new beneficial bacteria. I really recommend you try it out by buying a small bottle first before deciding to make your own: if you love it, you'll want to get your hands on more!

Buying kefir

You can now buy ready-made dairy or coconut kefir in larger supermarkets and health-food stores. I like Bio-tiful and Nourish in the UK. Look at the labels to get an idea of which strains of bacteria may be inside: the more the merrier.

You can buy plain versions, which can be used in sweet and savoury drinks and recipes. Or there are flavoured versions which are more like a traditional drinking yogurt.

If you have shops selling Polish or Eastern European products nearby, you may also find dairy kefir there, and often at a lower price as kefir is very popular in those countries. However, they may be a little sourer than the versions which have been developed to suit local tastes, which is why I recommend a more 'mainstream' version first.

Our panel included people living in South Africa and the Middle East, and they discovered traditional drinks with very similar profiles and potential benefits – laban and amasi. So do look for fermented milk products in your local area: it's fascinating to see that these drinks which are now becoming 'trendy' have been part of the food culture for centuries, all over the world. The knowledge of the benefits to the body and digestion has been passed down for generations.

Making kefir at home

Kefir is made from a 'scoby' – a symbiotic culture of bacteria and yeast. They're known as kefir 'grains'; but they actually look like either small jelly crystals, or, in the case of dairy kefir, tiny cauliflowers.

You can't create a scoby from scratch, but you can get it from some health-food shops or websites like Amazon. They need to go into milk at once, so don't order when you're about to go on holiday. Suppliers always send instructions, but here are my tips.

The basic method for home-made kefir

Kefir is made by mixing the scoby with cow's milk or goat's milk and letting it sit at room temperature in a lightly covered jar until the scoby ferments the sugars in the milk (lactose) and produces kefir. The speed of fermentation – and how sour the drink goes – depends on the weather, room temperature and the quantity of milk you add – if it's very warm and you don't add much milk, the drink will sour very quickly.

1. Weigh the scoby and add milk accordingly – in summer, add 200–250ml milk to every 5g or 1 tsp of scoby (use less milk in the winter: start with 150ml and watch closely to judge how quickly the milk ferments at the temperature in *your* house). Over time, the scoby will grow, so weigh it every time to ensure you're getting the proportion right.
2. Add to a large glass jar and cover loosely. Leave at room temperature but out of direct sunlight.
3. Check the appearance and taste after 18–24 hours – you can leave it a little longer in winter. The liquid will start to separate into curds and whey – the longer you leave it, the sourer it becomes, with more 'fizz'.
4. Once it's the right flavour for you, drain the liquid into a jug or bowl through a fine plastic sieve. The liquid is your kefir, ready for storing in a bottle or jar in the fridge

(which drastically slows, but doesn't completely stop fermentation). Use within 5 days.

5. The grains left in the sieve can be re-used straight away to make more kefir. As time goes on, they grow in size so you can make more, or give the grains to a friend.

Top tips

- Use whole milk, at least some of the time, as the scoby does better with it. With some scobies, you can also use coconut milk, but check with the company you're ordering from as they vary.
- I like to use organic milk – the money I'm saving on buying ready-made kefir means it is still good value with organic milk.
- Use your kefir in sweet or savoury dishes as you might use yogurt, but if you heat it, do so quite gently, and don't boil or you'll destroy the bacteria.
- If you're going away, place your scoby in a jar or plastic container, top up the jar with whole milk, cover and refrigerate for up to two weeks. The first batch you make after the break may be sourer – if so, discard, rinse scoby in filtered water in the sieve, and start again.
- If you've allowed to the mix to separate completely, and the liquid has gone grey, discard, rinse scoby in filtered water in the sieve, and start again.

The first time I tried kefir I must have had a bad batch as it was lumpy and curdled, but never having had kefir before I assumed that was just what it was like (particularly having heard it is an acquired taste for some). Speaking to others in our Dirty Diet group, I realised I may have just been unlucky and tried a different brand. I am so glad I did as I love it now!

Kim

Sourdough bread

Sourdough bread is made using a 'starter' culture, developed from water, flour and the naturally occurring yeasts in the flour. It has additional benefits to the other probiotics – it's not just about the effect the microbes have in your body, but also the effect they have on the flour that goes into your bread. The long proving time allows the bacteria (particularly Lactobacillus) in the 'starter' to begin digesting the grains. This makes the bread, once baked, much easier to digest, particularly for people with gluten sensitivity or IBS (though it's important to note that people with coeliac disease, a highly damaging auto-immune reaction to gluten, should still avoid sourdough and all wheat breads).

A lot of factory-made bread, including some supermarket sourdough, is made with commercial yeasts, and using the Chorleywood method, which speeds up the process. But speed isn't necessarily a good thing when it comes to food.

As well as being more digestible for some people, sourdough tastes fantastic, has a slightly chewier texture, and lasts much longer than commercially yeasted breads. It also makes great toast.

Buying sourdough

If you have a bakery nearby that does sourdough, ask them about their starter to make sure it's the real deal – in many cases they'll have had the same starter for years. Sourdough is more expensive to buy than most other bread because it takes much longer to make but, as I mentioned, it also keeps longer.

If you're buying from a supermarket, read the label – some will contain commercial yeast (listed as 'yeast') which means the bread has not had the long proving time, meaning the digestive benefits will not be present.

It's important to note that, unlike the other foods in this section, bread isn't really 'probiotic' when you eat it, because the high temperature of baking kills off the good bacteria. But you do get the benefits of the work they've done before baking!

Making sourdough at home

You'll need to spend a little time creating a starter from flour and water over several days. A starter takes wild yeasts from the flour and the air, and takes the place of commercial yeast in your bread dough. A good starter can last decades, as you reuse it over and over. Once your starter is thriving, it can be kept in the fridge and 'fed' once a week.

Your home-made sourdough 'starter'

Making a starter doesn't require anything fancy, just flour and water. It's not a quick process – you can't hurry it up or predict quite how it'll go – but have a little faith and patience, and you too could create something from (almost) nothing.

You will need:

Flour – rye and/or organic stoneground makes the most 'active' starter, but you can use any strong bread flour

Water – ideally filtered through a basic jug filter

A large glass or plastic bowl or container (I use a plastic box)

A cover that allows wild yeasts/bacteria in but not insects, which can be drawn by the fermentation. You can use a clean tea towel, muslin, a coffee filter, a disposable shower cap, or a sieve that fits over the bowl.

1. Combine 80g flour with 80ml water in your container. Leave on the kitchen counter at room temperature, but away from any other fermenting foods/open beer/ ripe fruit as you don't want the wrong bacteria in your starter. Cover loosely as above.

2. For the next 2 days, at around the same time, 'feed' your starter with another 75g flour and 75ml water and mix again, scraping down any flour from the sides of the container. Depending on temperature, it will begin to bubble and smell sour – or continue to add flour and water for up to 4 days in total until it does.*

3. Once the mixture is really beginning to bubble, discard HALF the starter (or give it to friends to start their own) and add another 75g flour and 75ml water. Repeat the discarding and refreshing each day for a total of 1 week to 10 days, until the mix seems stable and you're ready to bake (see recipe over).

---

* My starter exploded all over the kitchen on the morning of the fourth day, so do be aware that it can all happen quite suddenly!

When the sourdough is lively and bubbly, you can either carry on the discard/refresh every day (or a little less in colder temperatures: try every other day and adapt according to how fast it responds). Or you can store your starter, covered, in the fridge and feed it every week (it's a good idea to set an alarm on your phone or a reminder in your calendar!). This means it will stay usable, but won't need as much maintenance as one kept unrefrigerated.

To feed a refrigerated starter: take it out of the fridge once a week, discard a quarter of it and weigh the rest. Add the same weight of flour and water and leave for 24 hours. The starter should bubble back up and be ready to use to make a sponge/leaven that will then be usable the following day. Or simply put it back in the fridge till you need it or need to feed it again.

The basic method for home-made sourdough bread

Planning ahead is the key to this, because it takes longer for the bread to prove than with traditional yeasts.

Think of it as three main stages:

1. Making your 'leaven' or sponge from your starter (1–2 days before you bake)
2. Mixing the dough and proving overnight (the evening before you bake)
3. Baking in the morning.

The easiest way is to prep the leaven in the morning on day 1, make the dough in the evening on day 2 and let it prove overnight, then bake first thing on day 3.

Stage 1: Making your leaven

Mix 50ml of your starter with 50g of strong flour and 50ml water first thing in the morning. Leave it at room temperature, covered, till late afternoon/evening: ideally you want to go to stage 2 after 8–12 hours.

Stage 2: Mixing the dough and proving

You will need:

The leaven from stage 1

100g starter

500g strong bread flour (a mix of 400g white plus 100g wholegrain makes a good first loaf)

300ml filtered water

10g salt (ideally fine sea salt)

1. Mix together all the ingredients except for the salt in large bowl. Cover with a tea towel or clean shower cap and let it sit at room temperature for 1 to 2 hours.
2. The dough will be sticky – mix with your hands or a scraper in the bowl and tip onto the work surface and knead for around 10 minutes until the dough is more elastic.
3. Place back in the bowl (clean it out first if there are bits of dry flour on the sides) and allow to rise, ideally till it's

doubled in size: this can be 1–3 hours depending on how active the starter is, and the warmth of the room.

4. Turn out a second time and knead again – this stage is called 'knocking back', as the dough will become smaller again.

5. Line the bowl with a clean, flour-dusted tea towel and tip the dough into it. Let it rise again for an hour or so and, just before bed, place in the fridge overnight (if you find you love baking bread, invest in a proving basket/ banneton which gives a lovely circular pattern to the top of the bread).

Stage 3: Baking the bread

1. Next morning, set your oven to its highest temperature, preheat a baking sheet, and boil some water. Pour the boiling water into a small roasting tin at the bottom of the oven.

2. Flour the hot baking sheet and tip the dough out onto it (so the side that has been face-down is now face-up). Flour lightly and place in the oven.

3. After 10 minutes at the highest temperature, turn it down to around 200°C/220°C fan/400°F/Gas mark 6 and bake for another 25–30 minutes, until the loaf sounds hollow when you tap it.

4. Slide off the tray onto a wire rack and let it cool right down, as the baking is still happening and if you slice it straight away – tempting as it is – the bread will be soggy inside.

I've always loved sourdough – proper bread that you can really get your teeth into, and it lasts really well – but I didn't eat it much, because I avoided bread. Well, it's now back on the menu – my gut was right all along!

Timo

Fermented vegetables

Interest in fermented vegetables – like German sauerkraut and Korean kimchi – is soaring, and that's down to the possible benefits for your gut bacteria. Instead of using vinegar, these ferments use natural bacteria present in the vegetables and the environment to pre-digest the vegetables. This has two big benefits – first, they're easier for us to digest and, second, they're a great source of more friendly bacteria. The exact bacteria will depend on where the vegetables were fermented, and which were used, but they tend to include the same lactobacillus group as yogurt and kefir, even though no dairy is used. These produce lactic acid, which gives the tangy flavour and keeps the vegetables from going mouldy.

Buying fermented vegetables

Many of the factory-made krauts and kimchis have been pasteurised, and this process will kill off most or all of the good bacteria too. So look for krauts and kimchis kept in the chiller cabinets: you're most likely to find these in health-food shops or, again, in Polish or Eastern European delis. These will have a shorter shelf-life than pickles in jars or tins.

Fermenting at home

Making your own fermented vegetables is easy – and even therapeutic! – though, as with all ferments, the results will vary each time. If you're new to fermented foods, eat small portions at first. The fibre and probiotic content means your taste buds *and* gut bacteria may need time to get used to them!

Home-Made Fresh Apple and Cabbage Sauerkraut (with 100+ variations!)

This is a basic recipe that you can adapt with fresh veg including beetroot, carrot, chilli peppers, leeks and any whole seeds like cumin, coriander and mustard seed. I like to use a mix of cabbages – red cabbage gives the whole pickle a deep pink colour! It *is* salty, but that's what you need to get the liquids coming out of the veg.

Ingredients:

1 cooking apple

1kg firm cabbage, e.g. red, white or Chinese

2 tbsp sea salt

1 tsp black peppercorns

1 tsp caraway or fennel seeds (or other whole seed)

You'll also need:

A very large bowl

Plastic food bags, if you have sensitive skin (for the very de-stressing process of pounding and crushing the veg by hand)

Glass jar(s) for the pickle (I use a 1-litre Kilner jar while it's

fermenting, then transfer into smaller jars to refrigerate)
A mandoline – it looks like a straight grater and is very
sharp – makes incredibly quick work of slicing cabbage. I
bought a *Good Grips* one with a hand-guard from Amazon
to make pickling less labour intensive.

1. Wash your hands, the bowl, the jar(s) and slicing
   equipment in hot soapy water and rinse before use.
2. Grate the apple (skin still on but don't include the core)
   and finely slice or shred the cabbage (except the core) but
   keep back 1–2 large outer leaves to use later.
3. Layer the apple and cabbage in the bowl with salt sprinkled
   in between the layers. Use bare hands or place hands into
   the food bags like gloves, and firmly squeeze the salt into the
   veg for around 5 minutes, until they start to release liquid.
4. Leave for up to 15 minutes and repeat the massaging till
   the veg is reduced in size and there is plenty of liquid.
   Transfer the veg to a large jar, compacting it down as much
   as possible, pushing any air bubbles out* and ensuring
   that the veg is under the liquid. If there isn't enough liquid
   to completely cover the veg, you can add a little mineral
   water: add ¼ teaspoon sea salt to every 100ml and add to
   the jar.
5. Cover the veg with a spare cabbage leaf or two, followed
   by food-safe cling film. You can also fill a smaller jar with

---

* Fermentation is anaerobic so you don't want the veg to have any contact
with the air as it will make it go off. It's very rare, but if it does happen, it will
no longer smell sour, but very definitely 'off' or rotten. Discard the whole batch
and start again.

water and place on top, to make sure the veg stays under the liquid. Leave at room temperature for between 1–3 weeks: the warmer the weather, the faster it'll ferment.

6. Check every day to ensure veg are still submerged and to release any CO_2 that has built up during the fermentation process. After 7 days, begin to taste the veg – it will become sourer over time. Once it reaches the sourness you like, decant into smaller jars and store in the fridge.

Ingredient tips for fermented vegetables from Loving Foods

Faye and Mendel from Cheshire-based Loving Foods started producing raw, naturally cultured, fermented foods and drinks after using the products themselves to treat their IBS and eczema. Mendel is now trained as a nutritional therapist, and together they sell a variety of fermented foodstuffs: www.lovingfoods.co.uk . Here are their tips:

- Cabbage, radishes, beetroot and other roots and brassicas are particularly good to use as they ferment extremely well and keep for long periods.
- Ginger is another great ingredient. In addition to fermenting well, it has wonderful anti-inflammatory properties.
- Turmeric adds colour and flavour: the compounds in it are more easily absorbed when used with black pepper.
- Carrots are full of carotenoids, which are powerful antioxidants. Their sugar content also helps the fermentation process along so they also tend to be easy to ferment.

I had some spare red cabbage, so I thought I'd have a go. I was a bit dubious during the fermenting stage as it was bubbling away. However, after refrigerating it when it got to the right stage, I can honestly say it was worth it. Very tasty (although an acquired taste), with a lovely heat to it as I used chillies. If I've run out of kefir, it's a good back up to have. But it's also good with a salad too.

Jenni

A note on commercial 'bio' drinks, yogurts and other probiotic drinks

You can find more guidance on commercial probiotics in the supplements section on p. 320. In general, the small pots of probiotic drinks (e.g. Actimel or Yakult) or the probiotic yogurts (e.g. Activia) have single strains of specific bacteria. As our theme in this book is diversity, we prefer to use natural yogurts and kefir, but those products marketed as probiotic have been tested and found to be effective for specific issues, like constipation, or helping recovery from antibiotic-induced diarrhoea. However, they often contain sweeteners or added sugar, which we recommend not including in your diet.

You may also want to try **kombucha** – a fermented tea drink. Like water kefir, this is made with a scoby.

Kombucha does contain probiotics, but because it can attract less beneficial bacteria, the more commercial brands are usually heat-treated, which reduces the probiotic content. It also contains some caffeine – if you like it and enjoy it, then there may be some digestive benefits, but do keep an eye on the sugar content.

Choosing ready-made meals and prepared foods

Eating foods that haven't been over-processed is a key part of the Dirty Diet. But ready-made or partly prepared foods don't have to be unhealthy. They can be really handy when you're short of time or if you're at work – when you can't do any preparation except maybe putting something in the microwave, if you're lucky. Let's take a look at what our Dirty Dieters love to eat when they're in a hurry.

Before the Dirty Diet I would have been eating loads of meat and a few veggies, and usually only one type! Now it's four or five types of veggies and often no meat – I just don't need it! Another quick meal I have when I'm running in and then running out again is avocado on sourdough toast, with blue cheese or feta if I have calories available, with some cherry tomatoes and a salad on the side – quick to make and quick to eat. I've even made it into a sandwich to eat on the go!

Sarah

I have a few standbys now: salad with blue cheese and oil/balsamic dressing or home-made veg soup (I keep a stash in the freezer), or the Glorious brand of soups with a slice of sourdough.

Judith

Mine is a tray of roasting vegetables – a Mediterranean medley – with a sauce made from blue cheese and crème fraîche. It's absolutely delicious! I could eat it every day of the week.

Helen B

I have relied on COOK's single-portion calorie-controlled frozen meals, which are all under 400 calories (and most seem to be under 350 calories).

Bridget

All these dieters are enjoying success on the Dirty Diet – which shows the right prepared meals can be a godsend! But not all ready-made foods are created equal.

Tips for choosing good ready-made foods

- Read the label, including the small print and any national labelling system. For example, the UK traffic light system helps you identify the levels of fat, salt and sugar in products. Check portion size – a pack might serve 2, not 1, so will be higher in calories than you thought.
- Generally, the fewer – and more familiar – the ingredients listed the better.

- Don't dismiss frozen and canned. But, as for ready-made prepared meals, do the same checks as above on the labels.
- Avoid individual servings of fruit or veg (except those nature has packaged that way). This is an expensive way to eat raw ingredients that take little preparation. But with nuts or seeds, you *may* consider these if you want to get a sense of correct portion sizes. Try them for a week or so, then buy small containers and make up your own portions.

Prepared foods that can help on the Dirty Diet:

Soups from the chiller cabinet (and some canned soups too)

Look for those with lower salt content – the label on the front will show a traffic light warning and you should avoid those showing red. Vegetable and pulse-based soups will generally be more filling for fewer calories.

Prepared stir-fries or vegetables

These can be time savers – the chopping has been done for you, and if you are cooking for one, it saves buying larger veg that may go to waste. Also, you can now sometimes find ready-made 'courgetti' or sweet potato noodles. The downside is that these will lose some nutritional value as they're stored, and may not taste as fresh. But as Helen says:

Prepped veg is brilliant because it helps you maximise your overall intake of different veg. It's better to do it yourself but

this way really helps you – and your body – get used to trying
and using more delicious fresh produce in your meals.

You should still aim to add some protein – meat, fish, tofu or egg – and a simple sauce or marinade when cooking.

Prepared salads
The same considerations apply as to stir-fries and vegetables. Look for freshness through the packaging. Also, go for salads with a pot of dressing on the side: that way, they tend to be less soggy than if they're pre-dressed, and you also have a choice about how much of a calorific or sugary dressing to add.

Prepared sandwiches
Sandwiches, rolls and wraps are portable and tasty, so it's no wonder they're a lunchtime favourite. If possible, go to a deli or sandwich bar where you can choose your own filling – stacking up on fresh salad and protein-rich fillings, and choosing lower-calorie dressings or extras like mustard or even sauerkraut.

But shop-bought sandwiches do have the advantage of being calorie-counted – scrutinise the labels, as for ready-meals, and aim for wholegrain breads and leaner fillings.

Sushi
A tray of sushi can work out lower in calories than a sandwich, but the large amount of rice could make you sluggish. Choose dishes with good portions of protein-rich fish, egg or tofu, and eat alongside seeds or nuts, seaweed or edamame beans (which you can buy frozen).

Soy sauce is salty, so use sparingly.

Vegetable-based microwaveable meals

The prepared meals in clear pots that show visible pieces of veg are promoted as contributing to your five-a-day and are often around the 300–400 calorie mark. These may not be quite as nutritious as making your own, but they are often well balanced and easy to prepare. However, they can be more expensive, with a shorter shelf life than traditional microwave meals.

Cooked-chilled/frozen ready meals

These more traditional ready meals come in microwaveable or metallic trays, ready to be reheated. They can be useful, but recent scandals around the use of horsemeat in a small number of lasagnes show it's important to balance value with reliability of supplier.

Check the label and ingredients, and aim for dishes with vegetables high up in the list of ingredients, or serve alongside two portions of vegetables rather than chips.

Quiches, pizza and pasta dishes

These can make a quick lunch or supper, and though pastry is quite high in calories, an egg filling to a quiche or a vegetable-based pizza topping can be a decent basis for a meal. Serve with a large salad or extra veg.

Filled pasta is useful because it keeps for a week or two unopened in the fridge. I recommend adding fresh veg like green beans or young spinach to the cooking water to increase the veg content and, again, serve with a salad which fills at least half of your plate.

Eating out and takeaway guidance

I love eating out – where I live, in central Brighton on England's south coast, new places open every week and I can't wait to try them out with my partner or friends. So if you're like me, you won't want to stop eating out. And the good news is that the pattern of intermittent fasting accommodates that. But you always need to balance that with the need to consume fewer calories than you're using, if you're trying to lose weight.

Adapting your Blueprint to allow for eating out and takeaways as Bliss Moments

You can adapt your Blueprint to accommodate eating out within your plan. So, plan for eating a few more calories on the days you go out or get a delivery (while still making healthy choices!) – and reduce your intake on the days when you don't.

If you eat out or get a takeaway every night, though, be realistic: now may not be the time to undertake the Dirty Diet. But you can still increase the diversity in your diet, and ensure you include pro- and pre-biotics.

What to eat when eating out

I read endless articles about eating out during my decades of dieting, before starting to do 5:2. Generally, they recommended skipping bread and desserts, choosing lean cuts of meat, and asking for dressings and sauces on the side.

All of which *is* good advice. But it can take some of the enjoyment out of eating out – most of us with basic cooking skills can grill a chicken breast or sear a tuna steak and pop it on top of some salad at home. One of the pleasures of eating out is trying new things and eating fancier dishes than we usually have time to make at home.

Brilliant buffets – or beware?

Research shows that, perhaps unsurprisingly, we tend to take more from a buffet than we'd usually eat at home, and that the more variety there is, the more things we tend to take. Then, even if we're full, we find ourselves clearing our plates so we don't look like we took too much.

Yet buffets can be a good chance to make healthy choices:

- See if you can get as many of your seven-a-day if there's a salad bar.
- Try to build a colourful, beautiful plate that you imagine your healthiest friend enjoying, with veg, salad, nuts, seeds and a piece of protein the size of your hand (see more on this easy way to judge portion sizes on p. 317).
- Think with your microbiome – remember that each microbe has a different favourite veg or fruit, so aim to satisfy them all.

305

As an example, I did this recently at my favourite hotel in Greece. The buffet is incredible, and I decided to think with my microbiome (as well as my sweet tooth). So on my starters plate, I loaded up with:

- six different types of prepared salads, including ones in every colour;
- some fresh veg, including peppers, tomatoes and the darkest salad leaves I could see, plus some stalks of asparagus;
- a selection of nuts and seeds (a few of each);
- tzatziki, hummus and aubergine dips;
- a couple of different dressings, one with blue cheese and one with Greek olive oil;
- two different slices of yummy-looking bread.

I'd never have time to prepare all those things at home, and though it was certainly not a 'diet' meal, I could almost hear my friendly bacteria jumping for joy.

Top 'fast food' choices

I'm not going to claim that there's a magic takeaway out there that will help you lose weight. Many takeaways serve over-processed deep-fried food that doesn't tick any health boxes. But, if you can't resist the *occasional* takeout or delivery, you can make less damaging choices by doing some of the following:

- Select veg-based curries or yogurt-marinated meats like chicken tikka (*not* chicken tikka masala), or stir-fries with lots of seasonal veg.

- If you're having a pizza, or a pie, or chips, consider sharing the smallest portion with a friend or family member – and never, ever accept the offer to go super-size!
- Leave what you don't want – if the batter on your fish and chips is a bit too soggy, it's not worth the calories! Throw it away before you pick at it . . .
- Look beyond the obvious takeaways – Middle Eastern/Lebanese restaurants can offer delicious vegetable/pulse-based mezze, or Japanese food can be prepared in health-conscious ways.
- If you live in a city, you might even have a vegetarian takeaway or salad bar – I'm spoiled in Brighton, but brands like Leon or Itsu in the UK offer healthy choices.

Ever wondered what a dietitian does when she fancies a takeaway?

> **Helen says:** *I love a takeaway just as much as the next person – who wants to cook on a Friday night when you've had a busy week at work? A takeaway once a fortnight is nothing to feel bad about. But I have never liked greasy takeaways that leave you feeling over-full, sleepy and a bit grubby. My favourite takeaway, and the one that I suggest to my clients, is Thai – I order green papaya salad and prawn green curry, sharing this with my husband. We skim the fat off the curry and cook our own rice at home so we can control the portions better. I also love Vietnamese restaurants serving pho, which are noodle soups packed with fresh herbs and veggies.*

Now when I go to a restaurant, I don't obligate myself to have an appetiser plus an entrée plus a dessert just because that is the 'best deal'. I choose what is going to please me the most without making me feel bloated and sluggish for days. I am a lot more aware of how my body reacts to foods now.

Patricia

When eating out I now look at the veggie options first just to see if there's anything the Dirty Diet friendly (a recent trip to Café Rouge, a case in point, where I discovered their fabulous veg tagine), whereas before I wouldn't even bother to look at the vegetarian options. My tastes have changed so much – although I still love steak on occasions, the prospect of just steak and chips does not appeal in the same way any more. I'd much rather have a pile of veg or a really good salad than the chips . . . What has happened to me?!

Kim

THE DIRTY DIET IN ACTION:

'Health doesn't have to feel like self-denial
Louise, 46, cognitive behavioural therapist, West
Yorkshire, UK'

After 28 days: lost 8lbs (3.6kg), 40.3 BMI, down from 41.6, losing weight at last after failing at every other diet.

Louise says: This has been so enjoyable and illuminating – not like any other diet I have been on, and it doesn't need to feel like self-denial.

I am eating much healthier foods and smaller portions, I'm snacking less, I'm trying new recipes and, consequently, I am eating more fruit and veg. In general I'm focusing more on health than weight. A 16:8 approach really helped on Fast Days, as there were sufficient calories post-noon to feel like you're eating and having nice food, and I didn't really find missing breakfast much of an issue. I am planning on continuing with the plan in its entirety. The good thing is I can now just get back on the plan when I've had a minor blip – like going a couple of hundred calories over on a Plenty Day – without the guilt and consequent self-sabotage I've experienced on other diets.

I really don't feel I've been on a diet. I had almost concluded I was incapable of losing weight and this has shown me otherwise.

Health changes: Less moody, less acid reflux, more mentally alert.

Top tips: Fill in the Blueprint. I found it helpful to focus on where I was, where I was trying to get to, the potential obstacles, and my motivators.

Part 4:
Dirty for Life

Tools for living well and living 'dirty'

In this section, learn how to stay 'dirty for life', including:

- How to maintain after the four-week plan; including a simple way to stop calorie-counting for good;
- A guide to supplements;
- A look at how exercise helps with long-term weight maintenance;
- Guidance on how to keep a food diary to review and improve your diet further;
- You and Your Microbes: – how to look after yourself and your microbiome at different stages, from pregnancy to later life;
- Insights into the future of personalised diet and gut health, from 'transplants' to microbe prescriptions.

Dirty for life:

reaching your ideal weight and staying there

The Dirty Diet is designed as a plan for life – so once you've reached your target weight, keep going and still enjoy how good the DIRTY principles make you feel. But you can afford to be more relaxed about calorie-counting – hooray!

I advise you still to do one Fast Day a week for the health benefits, and as a reminder of your body's signals and its ability to be satisfied by less food. That helps with the biggest challenge – keeping the weight off after you've reached your goal.

The challenge to outwit your body's resistance to change

Everyone who has ever dieted knows that getting to that 'magic number' on the scales is only half the story. Staying there can be an even greater battle. The good – and bad news – is that it's not your 'fault'. It's your body that wants to take you back to square one.

Don't go changing . . .

The body is primed for survival. As we've seen, part of that is making sure that we don't starve, by laying down fat stores for periods of famine or shortage that, in our modern world, rarely come.

There's another principle at work, too: **homeostasis**. Or, your body's desire to keep things the same. This works in your favour most of the time – if you fall over and hurt yourself, or suffer an infection, the emergency systems are geared up to get you back to a healthy state.

But the body can interpret weight loss as an emergency too, and fight to get you back to 'normal', i.e. restore the weight you've worked so hard to lose.

Metabolism is one key factor – when we lose weight we already use fewer calories each day, because we're literally shifting less weight each day, which takes less energy.

A cycle of losing and gaining weight can also affect how we use energy long term. Experiments suggest this cycle might make our bodies more efficient – but that means we may find we put on weight even if we're following our TDEE as a guideline.

Plus, hormonal changes can increase our appetite so we really struggle to suppress the urge to eat more, and go back to our previous weight – which our body wants.

The Biggest Loser™ – back to square one

If you've ever watched *The Biggest Loser*™ – the TV show where people who are obese compete to lose weight, you'll have seen dramatic successes. The contestants' bodies, diets and health are transformed by intensive exercise, food and psychological coaching. But what happens when they go home?

The answers are depressing, and also familiar for anyone who has 'yoyo-ed'. Not only did most of the contestants regain most or all of the weight they lost, metabolic testing showed their energy use had slowed right down. Their bodies seem to be actively trying to get them to put the weight back on. And, eventually, they get tired of resisting the huge mental effort of sticking to an intense diet and exercise programme all the time.

Mind over matter

The good news is that with the Dirty Diet, you're avoiding many of the factors that make dieting difficult to stick to for life.

- No food is banned, so you're not having to deny yourself day after day, year after year.
- You're increasing your fibre and fresh produce consumption, which are both features of diets that promote healthy weight.
- Intermittent fasting may protect against metabolic slowdown more than conventional day in, day out dieting.

What to do after you reach your goal

First of all, celebrate! It's a fantastic achievement. Now, plan the next stage of your healthy life.

- Go through the Blueprint chapter again to plan the next stage of your healthy life.

- In particular, recalculate your TDEE: being a lower weight will also lower your TDEE, so you may want to increase activity levels or exercise to compensate (see p. 84 for guidance).
- Review how the principles will fit you in the future:

Diverse diet – This will be easy to maintain now it's a habit – keep the vegetable and fruit count high.

Intermittent fasting – We recommend one Fast Day per week, perhaps at a slightly higher calorie limit than before, but no more than 800 calories. You'll keep the benefits of intermittent fasting, and stay aware of how smaller meals can help you feel satisfied and energised.

Restoring gut health – Maintain your probiotic and prebiotic intakes.

Training in healthier habits – Once one habit becomes second nature, try a new one – whether it's being more active or experimenting with new foods.

You – It's still all about your needs and goals, so set new ones, and don't forget to work in your Bliss Moments.

What about calorie counting?

We talked about how calorie counting can be a real education in how much you're eating without realising, even if it's a bit tedious. But now you're maintaining – and have probably learned a lot about healthy portion sizes – here's a simpler alternative approach . . .

Down with calorie counting – up with the High Five approach

You can get a good sense of correct portion size by using your hand! Hands are good because they're – ahem – on hand, and their size varies between individuals, so it's a smart indicator of the size of different kinds of food you should be eating in your regular main meals.

- Protein (meat, fish, tofu, eggs): a piece the size of the middle of your palm
- Carbohydrates, e.g. cooked rice or pasta (ideally wholegrain and/or heated and cooked): the size of your fist
- Fat, e.g. butter or oil: a portion the size of the top part of your thumb (above the knuckle)
- Vegetables: have as many portions as you like! I always aim for diversity rather than large portions of a single veg – which also helps to balance out any calorie variations, as some vegetables are more energy-dense than others. A portion the size of your fist or slightly larger is fine.

Obviously, there will be times when you don't stick to these guidelines – eating out, or at celebrations. But they're a good, totally personalised indicator of what you need.

Supplements

The world of vitamins, supplements and branded 'superfoods' can be overwhelming, and it can be hard to tell the genuinely helpful from the snake oil. The supplements industry in the UK alone is worth an estimated £420 million.

Supplements can be beneficial, but if claims look too good to be true, they probably are. Check with NHS Choices, your GP or a dietitian if you're considering a supplement for a specific condition.

Multivitamins and minerals

Our meal plans are well balanced, but as you're eating less on a Fast Day, we recommend taking a multivitamin and mineral supplement on these days. It's best not to mega-dose on vitamins, but to go for a broad-spectrum multivitamin and mineral supplement from a reputable brand such as Centrum Advance or Sanatogen Complete. If this is taken with your main meal that day it will be best absorbed along with the nutrients in the food you are eating.

Vitamin D

This vitamin is important for bones, muscles and teeth. It is contained in food, but the body also produces it in response to sunlight on bare skin. In recent years, there's been increasing attention on how difficult it can be for people living in the northernmost countries (including the UK) to get enough during the winter months, so the current NHS advice is that adults can take up to 10mcg of vitamin D a day from October to March. In addition, if you have darker skin, or spend most of your time indoors, your body may not produce enough of the vitamin, and you could consider taking the supplement all year round.

Vegans and vegetarians

A well-balanced vegetarian or vegan diet may provide more vitamins and minerals than a poor diet that contains meat. However, you should consider vitamin B12 if you don't eat dairy produce, or eat very little. In addition, you could consider a multi-vitamin that ensures sufficient zinc, calcium and iron (a vegan diet can provide all of these, but may not always deliver enough).

Mega-doses of vitamins

Apart from B12 for those who don't eat many or any animal products, we generally don't recommend specific vitamins – certainly not in the 'mega-doses' sold online or in some stores. At best, you may be losing most of the vitamins in your urine – at worst, there can be undesirable effects long term.

There may be some occasions when a single vitamin or compound might help – for example, some women find magnesium helps with pre-menstrual symptoms. But do your research to avoid wasting money.

Probiotics

You'll know we are very keen on probiotics in food form, including kefir and fermented vegetables. But what about the capsules, pills or the special drinks marketed specifically for their probiotic contents?

There is evidence of probiotic supplements working for people with:

- diarrhoea from antibiotic use;
- diarrhoea from an infection;
- irritable bowel syndrome;
- lactose intolerance;
- constipation;
- ulcerative colitis.

The supplements' labels will identify the strains of bacteria and also how many 'colony forming units' they contain – i.e. the number of bacterial cells that are capable of dividing and then taking up residence in your gut. These tend to be impressive numbers, in the millions or billions. However, there are questions around this boom in probiotic supplements:

- Are the manufacturers being honest about the contents?
- How many of the bacteria will survive the processing and the transport between the manufacturers and the store and on to your home?
- Once at home, do they need to be refrigerated to survive?

- Crucially, will they survive the journey from your mouth to the gut, especially when they pass through the highly acidic environment of the stomach?

Helen says: For probiotics to work well they must be taken correctly. I advocate following the practical tips for taking probiotics from the British Dietetic Association. First you need to find the right strain that has been shown to work for your condition: see the table over the page. Then check that the quantity of probiotics in your supplement will be enough to be of benefit: take at least 100 million cfu per day, or check the suggested dose on the bottle as you may need more. Also, check the label to be sure the supplement has not expired, and for whether it needs to be kept in the fridge or not. You'll need to take it daily (and not with hot drinks, don't kill it off before it reaches your intestines!), and for conditions such as IBS take it daily for four weeks to give it a chance to work.

Generally, it's good to look for a probiotic supplement that combines several different strains. We're not yet at the stage where we can know exactly which strain might benefit each person individually, so taking one with a mix of different bacteria increases your chances of hitting the microbiome jackpot!

Here are some of the strains of bacteria that have been identified as useful:

Condition	Strain	Suggested product
Irritable bowel syndrome (IBS)	Bifidobacterium infantis 35624	Alflorex, Align, or OptiBac (capsules)
	Bifidobacterium breve, Bifidobacterium longum, Bifidobacterium infantis, Lactobacillus acidophilus, Lactobacillus plantarum, Lactobacillus paracasei, Lactobacillus bulgaricus and Streptococcus thermophilus	VSL #3 (sachet) Vivomixx (sachet or capsules)
	Lactobacillus rhamnosus GG (LGG)	OptiBac, Culturelle (capsules)
Prevent antibiotic-associated diarrhoea (take within 24 hours of starting antibiotic)	Lactobacillus rhamnosus GG (LGG)	OptiBac, Culturelle (capsules)
	Lactobacillus casei DN-114001	Actimel, Danactive (fermented milk)
	Lactobacillus acidophilus CL 1285 and Lactobacillus casei LBC80R	Bio-K (fermented milk)
	Saccharomyces boulardii	Florastor(capsule), OptiBac

Diarrhoea (start taking within 24hrs of start of diarrhoea)	Lactobacillus rhamnosus GG (LGG)	OptiBac, Culturelle (capsules)
	Saccharomyces boulardii	Florastor(capsule), OptiBac
Lactose Intolerance	Lactobacillus bulgaricus and Streptococcus thermophilus	Found in most yogurts
Constipation	Bifidobacterium lactis DN-173010	Activia (yogurt)
Ulcerative Colitis	E. Coli Nissle 1917	Mutaflor (capsule)
	Blend of 8 strains. See IBS above.	VSL #3 (sachet) Vivomixx (sachet or capsules)

Table © EatRight Ontario Updated to reflect UK probiotic brands available at the time of writing.

To see the official NHS advice (which is thorough but can be a little slow to reflect new findings), go to: www.nhs.uk/Conditions/probiotics/Pages/Introduction.aspx.

And for fascinating research from across this field, see the links in the Resources section (p. 347).

Inulin and fibre supplements

Inulin is a form of fibre found in many of the vegetables we recommend in the Dirty Diet, including onions, leeks, artichokes and asparagus. But it can also be consumed as a supplement, usually processed from chicory root, and turned into a powder which can be diluted with water or mixed into foods, to give you a boost.

Various studies have shown that inulin may help with constipation and aid weight loss, with potential further health benefits due to the gut bacteria fermenting inulin and producing the short-chain fatty acid butyrate (see p. 57). However, there is a downside, especially if you experience IBS symptoms. You can suffer increased bloating or abdominal pain and diarrhoea.

> **Helen says:** *Inulin and FOS (fructooligosaccharides) are the most well-known prebiotics, which means they support growth of good bacteria in your colon. An effective intake is at least 10g daily, so if taking as a supplement or fortified within food, check the label or ingredient list for amounts.*

Psyllium husks have been on the market for some years, and bulk out quickly. They can help with constipation, but, again, may lead to bloating, cramping and wind. It is best to get enough fibre through foods in your diet, but if this is not possible fibre supplements such as psyllium husks can help. Take with plenty of extra fluids. If taking for laxative purposes, consult your GP.

Omega 3 and 6 fatty acids

Omega 6 (linoleic acid) and omega 3 (alpha-linoleic acid) can't be produced by the body but are essential fatty acids, needed for good health. Having the balance of the two is also important, and getting it right can be difficult. If you eat oily fish like salmon, this will provide some omega 3, but you may want to consider fish oil or flaxseed supplements. Food sources include ground flaxseeds or chia seeds, which you can sprinkle on yogurt or savoury dishes; rapeseed oil in dressings or cooking; or whole walnuts.

Superfood supplements and herbs

Again, it can be hard to tell the difference between herbal supplements that may have been taken for centuries with apparent good results and hyped-up pills promising the earth but delivering little more than profit for the makers.

'Herbal' supplements sound innocent, but remedies like St John's wort – traditionally used in some countries to treat mild depression – can have side effects or interfere with conventional medication.

Newer supplements like curcumin – taken by those wanting to capitalise on the research showing potentially powerful antioxidant properties of the spice turmeric – may have potential, but their effects are unproven in human studies.

Aloe vera drinks, raspberry ketones, and other supposed diet or digestive aids that are sold by multilevel marketing companies are not recommended.

Generally, we suggest that you should focus on whole foods to get the full health benefits of spices, or produce. We can't be certain that curcumin on its own, for example, is giving the same benefits as turmeric used in food. A bowl of raspberries or a curry rich in turmeric are certainly tastier and cheaper.

Exercise and weight loss

Exercise is great for all-round health. It's not *essential* for weight loss – so if you are restricted in how much you can move, you can still make big health improvements. But being active helps to use energy and can increase our muscle mass, which raises metabolism. It's also great for flexibility. Plus, weight-bearing exercise, including walking and running, helps with bone density, which matters as we age.

The NHS advises at least 30 minutes of exercise – activity that leaves us slightly out of breath but still able to carry on a conversation – five times per week.

However, there's some evidence that extra exercise or activity may make us want to eat more to compensate. And exercise itself often burns fewer calories than you expect. So do take care not to 'eat back' your calories: those are already taken into account in your TDEE when you pick your activity level as part of the calculation.

Organised exercise vs being more active day-to-day

Over the last 50 years, we've seen obesity rise, despite huge growth in the exercise sector, from gyms to DVDs and personal trainers. We tend to think of previous generations walking or running long distances. In many cases, that wouldn't explain the weight difference: it's more the case that everyday life itself was more active, from our work to our home lives. Sedentary lives are dangerous!

One study by researchers at Leicester and Loughborough universities in the UK analysed data from 800,000 people and concluded that the risks of premature death, especially from diabetes, were much higher in people who sat or lay down the most. Another university team found a connection between hours spent inactive and the likelihood of disability over the age of 60.

The best approach is probably to combine both. So in an ideal world, you will do an enjoyable activity/exercise that raises the heart rate and challenges the muscles *and* try to be more active day-to-day.

Working activity into your life

NEAT stands for non-exercise activity thermogenesis, and means all the activities you do that aren't intended as 'exercise' but still consume energy (and burn calories!). It's about the activities – even fidgeting – you do that you don't think of as exercise, but do raise your heart rate and move your muscles. Include more of the following in your daily life and you'll burn more calories and feel more energetic:

- walking to a shop further away to buy your lunch;
- taking the stairs instead of the lift;
- having business meetings standing up or walking;
- walking on the spot while watching TV;
- cleaning, ironing, cooking that bit faster;
- standing up and having a really good stretch of all your muscles when you've been sitting for too long.

Personally, I do go to the gym, but not because it's a huge factor in weight loss. It's more because I like how it makes me feel. Plus working my heart a bit harder is good for my overall cardiovascular health.

But I also try to move more every day. My job, like so many people's, is sedentary. But I have a Fitbit that buzzes every hour if I haven't done enough moving around. It might seem trivial, but it's a good reminder to me to move as I'm designed to – I take a walk around the house, have a stretch or take the dog round the block. It helps mentally, too. And as I get older, I'm more aware of the need to stay flexible, so I stretch and do Pilates as well.

How to keep a
two-day food diary

As we said in the Blueprint chapter, keeping a two-day food diary can give you lots of insight into how food might affect your health. You can use this as a baseline for how you feel from week to week, and to review how your diet is improving.

You can either use apps that help you to monitor your intake and any health symptoms – or you can simply use a notebook to keep a food diary.

Using apps to monitor your food intake and any symptoms

MyFitnessPal or, better still, MySymptoms both have free versions for Android and iPhone, which will help you monitor:

- Food intake;
- Mood/triggers;
- Symptoms;
- Digestion – bowel motions, frequency, any discomfort.

If you have symptoms you suspect relate to food, you may want to keep going with a tracker for longer to track changes and improvements, or possible intolerances.

Using a notebook to monitor your food intake and any symptoms

Get a small notebook you can carry around with you and note:

- Time of eating;
- What you ate/quantities;
- Mood and symptoms before, during and after food; score symptoms 0–5 (where 5 is the worst);
- Any symptoms you note during the day, whether they seem associated with food or not;
- Sleep patterns.

Analysing your diary

Helen uses food diaries with her clients to help them see patterns and make changes. They're best used as a short-term measure – doing this all the time could lead to obsessive eating. Here are her tips:

Food diaries are a fantastic tool for gaining insight into your eating habits. All of us suffer from some degree of 'food amnesia', but if we record by pen, photo or app every single thing we eat or drink during the day, it does three things: it helps us realise exactly what we are eating, why we are eating it, and how it makes us feel (how our bodies respond to that food). It can also help us to think twice about what is about to pass our lips, and so help motivation when making dietary changes.

Look for patterns. Are you a snacker? Are your portion sizes out of control? What are you doing well? Try and pick out a couple of points from your food diary that are positive and you would like to continue, and a couple of aspects you could improve.

A food diary could highlight several things that a registered dietitian can support you with. For example, are you experiencing regular bloating, pain, gas and/or change in bowel habit in relation to specific foods? Are you eating for emotional reasons rather than hunger and feel you cannot control this? For access to a NHS dietitian you can phone your local dietetic department to see if they offer a self-referral system, or seek a referral from your GP. Alternatively, in the UK your local private dietitian can be located using: freelancedietitians.org

You and your microbes – friends for life

The changes that have helped restore your gut health will help weight maintenance *and* general health as well as your digestion.

But your age and lifestyle also alter your microbiome.

Birth and breastfeeding

The microbes in a pregnant woman's vagina change as labour approaches – it's thought the changes encourage the right balance of bacteria which the baby encounters as it travels down the birth canal. Because an infant has no gut bacteria while it's in the womb, the microbes in the vagina are the first the baby encounters that will help it develop a healthy immune system. Babies who've been born vaginally have different gut microbes to those born by Caesarean section. This may affect their future weight gain, immunity and other health issues.

Breastfeeding also helps establish the microbes that encourage health and growth.

Of course, you can't do anything about your own birth and early life, but if you're planning to have children, it's useful to know that being born vaginally and then being breastfed gives a baby's gut microbiome the best possible start (as well as the many other benefits breastfeeding has).

Antibiotics

Antibiotics can be lifesavers, wiping out dangerous bacteria and curing infections and diseases. However, many can be very indiscriminate – they wipe out the good as well as the bad bacteria, which is why you often get diarrhoea when you take a course.

No one would suggest that you shouldn't take life-saving drugs. But these guidelines can help you during and after illness or infection.

- Don't go to the doctor expecting antibiotics for every illness – many are caused by viruses, so antibiotics will have no effect. Doctors have also been advised to prescribe fewer courses, because the dangerous bacteria are becoming resistant to antibiotics, making them less effective.
- If you are taking antibiotics, taking probiotics at the same time can reduce the side-effects, including diarrhoea. This has been proven with the probiotics listed in the table on p. 322.
- Carry on with yogurts, kefir or branded probiotics after finishing the antibiotic course, to help repopulate your gut with the good bacteria.

Antibacterial sprays, hand gels and wipes

These have become more common in the last few years. We're encouraged to wipe out all bacteria in our home – some ads claim to wipe out 99.9% of all bugs – using sprays and wipes. Outside the home, we can use antibacterial gels to wipe out the bugs on our skin.

But as you'll know from reading this book, many bacteria are *helpful* – and those sprays and gels don't discriminate between the good and the bad. The danger is that when you wipe out the good, the bad bacteria on your skin return in greater numbers and cause infections or irritation. One common antibacterial ingredient has been banned from hand soaps in the USA due to these concerns.

In the home, the same applies. We also don't know the effect on younger family members, whose microbiomes – those in the gut but also on the skin and in other locations – are still developing. The cleansers can also help the bad bacteria become more resistant. Of course, if you're travelling with no access to water, the gel cleansers can be useful before eating or after using the toilet. But for regular use:

- Choose household cleaning products that don't boast antibacterial properties. Most will still clean. If there's a tummy bug or other illness going around, swap to antibacterial if you like, till everyone is well, then go back to a standard product.
- Wash your hands instead of using antibacterial gel. Hand-washing removes bacteria *and* viruses without changing the overall balance. Wash for at least 20 seconds, ensuring you get to every part of the hands.

Later life – diversity becomes even more important

As we age, our gut microbiome gradually becomes less diverse, which is not good for our overall health. The changes can be associated with constipation and more inflammation. Other microbe-rich environments – like in our mouth – are also affected by losing teeth or not producing as much saliva too.

Maintaining a diverse diet becomes more important as we age: maintaining a healthy gut microbiome may even keep us feeling and looking younger. Research with older people in Ireland shows it's particularly important for those in residential care, as their diets and therefore microbiomes can become more limited than people living in their own homes.

- Our metabolism changes as we get older – we need less energy, partly because our muscle mass goes down. So eating more lower-calorie vegetables and fruit – lots of variety too, of course – makes sense for your weight and your gut.
- Include those fermented foods including the pickled veg and kefir or yogurt.
- Include lots of prebiotic foods to nurture the gut bacteria you already have – fibre, oats, nuts and the other foods we listed in the table on p. 271 onwards.
- Make more effort to try different foods and flavours – our appetite can suffer as we get older, so ensure you're keeping your food interesting and varied.

Testing your microbiome

Many of us will be curious about what's happening in our own microbiome, and how we compare with other people around the world. For this book, I attempted to have two samples tested, with inconclusive results.

The American and British Gut projects are exciting and ambitious, aiming to 'map' as many people's gut microbiomes as possible. As they are non-profit scientific studies, you're asked to make a financial donation to the research, which then entitles you to have your own microbiome sequenced by sending back samples. These can include stool samples to measure gut microbes, as well as samples from the mouth, skin or other locations in the body. However, only the gut microbe results will currently be reported back.

Because there are so many donations, there can also be a significant delay between sending your sample and seeing the results. In my case, it took around four months. The information isn't easy for a layperson to interpret but the results provide comparisons with other people with similar diets and backgrounds. It is also easy to download the full data, which could become more useful as knowledge grows.

There is a greater benefit to mapping a large population so that even if your individual results are slow to arrive, you could be making a contribution to longer-term research. British Gut points out that the field of personalised nutrition is fast-moving, so watch out for new developments!

Commercial tests are also coming on to the market, starting at about £125, but do check what information will be provided.

I paid for a test by Atlasbiomed.com which you can order direct as a consumer. The results were available online within six weeks, and were illustrated by attractive graphics and after an email exchange I was able to download more detailed data. When I asked microbiome scientists to review the information I was given, they were critical of the health predictions made, as their opinion is that nobody is in a position to do anything medically actionable with microbiome data at the moment.

Atlas Biomed responded by saying that their team is formed of geneticists, bioinformaticians, medical professionals, IT and business decelopment experts, with their work reviewed by an expert Scientific Advisory Board. The test analyses the DNA of the microbiome using 16s rRNA sequencing, with results compared to scientific papers. Users are given this information, plus food recommendations to improve their diet and promote their microbiome.

Follow your gut . . .

I'd say that right now, if you want to do the best for your microbiome, you may be better off spending your money on the healthy foods recommended in this book, rather than testing. But if you want to help with this exciting area of research, and gain a limited insight into your microbes, you may want to contribute to the gut projects in your own country. And do keep an eye on how the tests are evolving.

The future of microbiome, personalised weight loss and longevity research

We really are in the early stages of microbiome research, but the possibilities for human health are very exciting. These include:

- Gut microbiome testing for disease diagnosis or early warning: as knowledge increases about what the presence or absence of different microbes means, doctors may be able to diagnose diseases by analysing gut microbes. They could also potentially detect changes before a disease develops, offering early warning for conditions including type 2 diabetes.
- Probiotics for prevention or treatment: as well as diagnosing disease, it's likely that doctors will be able to use bacteria and other microbes to treat conditions. Probiotics have already been used to prevent diarrhoea, and to treat various digestive conditions.
- Faecal or 'poo' transplants: these have already been used with patients suffering from a very difficult-to-treat

infection that can arise in hospitals (*C. difficile*). But taking faeces from healthy donors and giving it to people with a range of other conditions may become more common. These transplants have also been shown to affect weight, with donations from leaner people having a positive effect on both obese patients and those with type 2 diabetes. However, the intervention can also have the opposite effect, with weight gain *after* transplant.

• Personalised diets based on our gut bacteria: a slightly less drastic option than transplants could be very personalised diets based on our current microbiome balance, designed to improve these and our metabolism through specific foods.

I asked Imperial College scientist Dr Lesley Hoyles about her predictions for the next decade of microbiome research. This is what she said:

> *We've already seen that microbiome composition can be used to predict how individuals will respond to different dietary challenges; gut microbes modify the effects of some cardiac and diabetes medications, and the diversity of our gut microbiome influences responsiveness to certain cancer therapies. These findings make it clear microbiome-based precision medicine is no longer a pipe dream.*
>
> *The future of microbiome research is very exciting. Basic science will answer, for example, the following: what is a healthy microbiome? How does your healthy microbiome differ from somebody else's? Is it the microbiome that causes*

disease, or is what we're doing to ourselves – and by extension to the microbiome – causing disease? How do we restore environmental conditions in the gut so that the beneficial microbes can re-establish their populations? How do the metabolites – chemicals – our microbiome produces affect our health, and can these be manipulated to benefit our health?

Ultimately, we will be able to predict from biomarkers in your metabolome, immune system and/or microbiome how you will respond to different foods or drugs, and which will provide the greatest health benefit to you – and only you.

To find out more, go to thedirty-diet.com where I've interviewed Lesley and other people about their work in this field. I also really recommend reading some of the brilliant books published on the topic. See the Resources section for more.

RESOURCES

Calorie counts, protein and veg portions of Dirty Diet meals

Breakfasts and Brunches	Protein (grams)	Veg portions	Cals
Portobello Mushroom Rarebit with Oven-Baked Tomatoes	16	2	280
Butter Bean Puttanesca with a Baked Egg	18	2	286
Greek Yogurt Fruit Sundae with Choc-Cherry Granola	9.7	2	294
Choc-Cherry Granola	2.4	0	104
Avocado Toast with Feta, Lime and Chilli	12.7	1.5	322
Waldorf Muffin (with 1 small apple and 20g blue cheese)	7.4 per muffin, 11.4g with apple and cheese	1	293
Sweet Potato Bubble and Squeak Mash with Blue Cheese/Horseradish Sauce	9	3	289
Fuss-Free Eggs Florentine/ Benedict/Royale	14–18	0–1	300–325

Overnight Power Oats with Fruit and Crunchy Nuts	up to 9	2	260–300
Heart-Warmer Porridge with Banana, Cinnamon and Pecans	7	1	306
Mexican Tomato Scramble on Toast	17–19	1	308–318

Soups and Light Meals	Protein (grams)	Veg portions	Cals
Mexican Smoky Bean Soup with Kefir Swirl	7	3	142
Green Star Minestrone with Pesto	9	2	153
Chickpea and Leek soup with Blue Cheese	8.4	2	144–170
Tomato and Strawberry Gazpacho with Egg or Seeds	4.3–6.2	3	145–150
Pumpkin and Lentil Soup with Herb-Infused Olive Oil	5.4	2	153
Quick-as-a-Flash Cauliflower and Broccoli Tabbouleh	7	3	131
Hot Artichoke and Pepper Spread with Mozzarella on Sourdough	7.5	1	137
Egg Pancake with Quick-Blistered Veg	10	1.5	147
Wedge Salad with Blue Cheese Dressing	6	2	120
Pink Tzatziki with Super-Fast Chickpea Flatbread	8	1	177
Thyme and Sweet Pepper Hummus with Crudités	7.2	3	153

Main dishes	Protein (grams)	Veg portions	Cals
Revved-Up Caesar Salad with Parmesan and Mustard Kefir Dressing	13/42	3	319
Blue Cheese, Leek and Potato Puff Bake	18	1	274
5-a-Day Vegetable and Paneer Balti	20	5	297
Chicken Dirty Rice with Spices and Bacon	21	2.5	345
Veggie Dirty Rice with Spices and Sausages	13	2	324
Mushroom and Tofu Chicken Stroganoff	20	3	303
Middle Eastern Spiced Bean Burgers with Halloumi, and Aubergine 'Buns'	19	3	310
Black Lentil Dal with Tomatoes and Creamy Kefir	18	1.5	276
Sweet Potato and Broad Bean Tortilla	16	1	293
Spicy Sesame Prawn/Tofu Noodle Salad with just veg	24.5	3 3	342 270
Punchy New Potato Salad with Egg and Pea Shoots	15	2	284
Sticky Ginger Chicken/Tofu with Turmeric Rice Noodles	50/18	3	473
Bacon, Bean and Spinach Risotto with White Wine Primavera Risotto Porcini Mushrooms and Leek Risotto	17.4 9.5 11	2 2.5 1.5	475 464 387

Filo Tart with Brie, Winter Veg and Bacon/Mushrooms	16/15	1	322/312
Filo Tart with Gruyère, Watercress and Roast Cherry Tomatoes plus salmon	16 19	1	315 342
Chilli-Spiked Vegetarian Cottage Pie	12.6	4	277
Beef, Mushroom and Cashew Stir Fry	27	4-5	342
Speedy Chicken Tikka Masala	37	4	320
Barley Pot with Balsamic and Mustard Roast Winter Roots	11	5	354
Hot Lamb Meatballs with Red Slaw and Cinna-Mint Drizzle	22	2	349
Mushroom and Black Bean Koftas with Cinna-Mint Drizzle, Red Slaw and Pitta Breads	13.4	3	268
Warm Puy Lentil Salad with Jewel Veg and Chilli Dressing	20	2.5	317
Smoked Salmon and Courgette Spaghetti with Creamy Watercress Sauce	24	2	392
Hot Devil Flatbread Pizza	14.3	2.5	325
Middle Eastern Veg Flatbread Pizza	17	4	322
Chicken Pasta Bake with Ricotta, Lemon and Vegetables	43	3	477
Sides	**Protein (grams)**	**Veg portions**	**Cals**
Refried Beans with White cheese and Coriander	6.4	1	107
Crunchy Sweet Slaw with Dill and Caraway	3	2	88

Kale Salad with Peas and Pesto Flavour	8.1	1.5	129
Purple Sprouting Broccoli with Romesco Sauce	6.8	2.5	154
Sweet Potato, Lime and Turmeric Wedges	1.8	1	139

Summer Berries with Kefir Cheesecake Topping	4.3	2	142
Little Kefir Parfait Shot	2.7	2	62
Dessert Black Berries Parfait Pot	5.7	2	155
Dark Chocolate Ginger and Apricot Truffles	0.6 each		27

Online resources, apps and recommended reading

Dirty Diet and gut health resources

The book's website www.thedirty-diet.com has downloads and great links to help you, including interviews and free, downloadable podcasts (audio recordings you can listen to on your phone, wherever you are) with tips on the topics covered in this book.

Other good sites for information about gut health and the microbiome include:

www.gutmicrobiotaforhealth.com (my favourite)
learn.genetics.utah.edu/content/microbiome
www.futurity.org/topic/microbiomes
loveyourtummy.org
www.mynewgut.eu

Books

I enjoyed all these books about gut health and the microbiome – it's such a fascinating area:

The Diet Myth: The Real Science Behind What We Eat by Tim Spector

Gut: The Inside Story of Our Body's Most Under-Rated Organ by Giulia Enders

10% Human: How Your Body's Microbes Hold the Key to Health and Happiness by Alanna Collen

Missing Microbes: How Killing Bacteria Creates Modern Plagues by Martin Blaser

Apps and food/calorie trackers

Myfitnesspal.com – free to use and well designed, but sometimes unreliable when data has been supplied by users.

Nutracheck.co.uk – I use this UK-based paid app/site (they offer a free seven-day trial). I like how it breaks down your intake into fat, protein and carbs, and it also connects with Fitbit.

Sparkpeople.com has exercise tips and videos, as well as calorie-counting information and food ideas.

MySymptoms app from skygazerlabs.com which Helen recommends if you want to keep a food diary to spot health issues.

Cultured food tips

There are dozens of websites devoted to dairy, coconut and water kefir, full of tips and research. I like culturesforhealth.com – and for bread, Vanessa Kimbell's inspiring sourdough.co.uk

Healthy recipes

You can find healthy recipes with ingredients and measurements suitable for your area at:

UK:
www.olivemagazine.com/recipes/healthy
www.bbcgoodfood.com/recipes/category/healthy
www.deliciousmagazine.co.uk/recipes/healthy-recipes

Australia/New Zealand:
www.taste.com.au/healthy
www.healthyfoodguide.com.au/recipes
www.bite.co.nz

USA :
www.eatingwell.com
recipes.heart.org
www.goodhousekeeping.com/food-recipes/healthy

THE DIRTY DIET IN ACTION
'A lesson in eating well and
the power of body and mind'

Alex, 34, resuscitation officer, Hampshire, UK

After 28 days: 14 lbs/6.5kg lost, 26 BMI, down from 28.2, dropped a dress size from size 14 to 12, sleeping better and less bloated.

Alex says: I love how I can eat what I like – food does not rule me, I rule it. I feel I have control and I am also happier, much less anxious and depressed.

I feel less bulky – I have tried Slimming World and Weight Watchers in the past, but find fasting works, as it teaches you about when you are actually hungry, and only eating when you require it, not because you feel you have to. I am going to carry on with the Dirty Diet as it works for me.

Health changes: I sleep much better and don't feel so bloated – my digestion is also much more regular. My blood sugar is more even and I don't get shaky if there's a delay eating.

Top tips: Don't get disheartened if you don't lose weight as you may still be losing inches. The body is a wonderful machine but it takes a little time to adjust. Also drink plenty of water: when I drink enough, I don't get hungry.

Last words from Kate and our very happy Dirty testers

Dear reader,

I want to thank you for reading the book – I hope you're on the way to achieving your goals and feeling healthier. I also want to thank the brilliant people who agreed to try out the Dirty Diet and share their thoughts.

So it seems right to end the book with *their* thoughts and comments.

Don't forget you can contact me via @katewritesbooks and @thedirtydiet on Twitter and also join our Facebook group for support and ideas – facebook.com/groups/thedirtydiet – plus stay up to date via thedirty-diet.com

Thanks so much for joining me on this journey – and if you enjoyed the book, do please let me know, or I'd be really grateful for a review of the book on Amazon to help other people discover the joy of living dirty. Meanwhile, let's end with the experiences of the people who've made it part of their lives.

Kate x

I'm definitely carrying on. It's the only diet that has made sense to me, and while it has made me a lot more conscious of what I'm eating, I don't feel obsessed by it or that I'm being a martyr. Love its flexibility. I also have more energy, which means I do more and burn more calories . . . not a vicious circle, but a virtuous one!

Bridget

For the first time in my life I have discovered a way of life and a way of eating that is not solely about losing weight. The Dirty Diet has taught me that the 'healthy' choices are often the tastiest and most satisfying choices; that eating well does not mean denying myself; and that if I am going to stay the size and weight I am now and want to be, then I must enjoy the lifestyle I am living. I can genuinely and honestly say that since beginning this way of life I am enjoying food more than ever before. I have discovered so many new foods and fantastic combinations of tastes that food has once again become a real pleasure rather than a guilty indulgence followed by regret and self-recrimination. The guilt has gone and I am loving food again!

Kim

I'll be carrying on. I find eating more veg so beneficial! And I'm sleeping better, plus my psoriasis, bowel movements and acid reflux have all improved.

Rose

I enjoyed the 'science' part of fasting, understanding the gut microbiome – it made a lot of sense to me and helped me understand the benefits of the diet from the start. For me, it's not a 'diet', it's a new way of life and changed eating habits. I'm carrying on – it's given me a refocus on my eating habits, and I am amazed how I've completely cut out snacking – I'm having two or three meals a day and I feel brilliant for it!

Holly

I'll definitely be carrying on. I feel better than I've felt over the last few years. My IBS has improved, even my other half has commented. I love being able to plan my meals for the week, as I then don't have to worry about it, but the plan is flexible enough that I can change my mind as well. Diet? What diet? This hasn't felt like a diet plan at all – it is a definite way of life. I'm over the moon with my losses – I can't believe how much better I feel in myself.

Jenni

What makes The Dirty Diet different, and better, is the emphasis on eating food that is not only good for you, but that TASTES good. There is no deprivation factor, and that is what you ALWAYS get on every other diet.

Patricia

They say it takes eight weeks to form a new habit . . .
Well, I have formed some great habits on the Dirty
Diet, including cutting out snacking, eating such a
variety of vegetables every day, and still no soft drinks
or takeaways! People comment on how I look but also
how positive I am. I have so much more energy! I have
dropped two sizes in my clothes, but most importantly of
all I feel happier than I have in years.

Sarah

General Index

antibiotics 52, 59–60, 62, 333

bacteria 29, 59, 60, 62, 64, 66, 121,
    122, 320, 321, 324, 332, 333,
    334, 335, 338, 339
    and Alzheimer's/mental health 61
    and diet 72
    and fasting 50
    and microbiome 53–5
    and probiotics 63, 65, 279, 280,
    281, 284–5, 287, 288, 289, 290,
    294–5, 298
    food influence on 31, 47
    in the gut 56–8
Body Mass Index (BMI) 84, 98, 99

calories 26, 27, 29, 30, 31, 32, 34, 36,
    41, 43, 44, 45, 74, 75, 76, 81,
    86, 94, 99, 104, 126–45, 281,
    302, 303, 304, 314, 326, 327
    calorie counter 270–8
    calorie-counting 146–7, 312,
    316–17
    calorie needs 83–4
    Dirty Diet meals 342–6
    and Fast Days 46, 100, 101, 102,
    316
    for meal plans 124, 126–45
    low-calorie foods 35, 39, 40, 301,
    302, 335
carbohydrates 64, 317
colitis, ulcerative 61, 320, 323

constipation 298, 320, 323, 324, 335

diarrhoea 59, 121, 122, 123, 298,
    320, 322–3
diets, failure of 74–6, 87
digestion 33, 34, 41, 49, 52, 55, 56,
    62, 121, 289,298, 325, 338
diverse diet 28–39, 316

eating disorders 86
energy needs 83
exercise 326–8

fasting days 26, 40, 41, 46–9, 99,
    100, 101, 102, 103, 108, 115,
    116, 147, 313, 316, 318, *see also*
    intermittent fasting
    meal planner 130, 136
fermented foods 335, *see*
    also vegetables
fibre supplements 323–4
food *see also* bacteria,
    meal plans
    diary 329–31
    eating out/takeaways 304–8
    for reduced fat, *see* 'smart
    harvesting'
    and gut microbes 63–5
    ready-made/prepared 299–303
    strategies for healthy eating 92–7
    to eat 31, 32, 33, 34, 35, 36, 71,
    72, 115–23, 317

gut 27, 29, 31, 33, 39, 44, 50, 75, 89, 116, 121, 122, 123, 281, 284, 294
restoring gut health 52–67, 316

healthy living 69–74, 316
herb supplements 325
homeostasis 314

Intermittent fasting (IF) 27, 39–52, 75, 100, 315, 316, 366
benefits of 39, 40–4
insulin 33, 43, 45, 47, 61, 63
inulin supplements 63, 67, 323–4
Irritable Bowel Syndrome (IBS) 121–2, 322

kefir, buying & making your own 284–8

lactose intolerance 32, 66, 280, 320

meal plans 124–45
metabolism 32, 34, 43, 44, 45, 314, 326, 335, 339
microbes 33, 54, 55, 56, 57–8, 59, 60–1, 62, 63, 65, 66, 67, 281, 284, 288, 332–7, 338, 339, 340
microbiome 31, 44, 53–4, 55, 56, 58, 59–63, 67, 69, 72, 75, 78, 109, 122, 305, 321, 332, 333, 334, 335, 336–7, 338–40
and disease 61
and mental health 61–2
and weight 60–1
motivation exercise 89–90
motivating factors 90–1

Omega 3 & 6 324–5

prebiotics 27, 52, 66–7, 125

probiotics 27, 44, 52, 62, 63, 65, 67, 125, 126, 132, 138, 142, 279–98, 320–1, 333, 338, 366
drinks 298
protein 28, 31, 34, 35, 40, 43, 56, 64, 65, 71, 72, 126, 132, 138, 142, 281, 302, 305, 317, 342–6

'smart harvesting' 27, 28, 30, 31–5, 116
sourdough, buying & making your own 288–94
superfood supplements 325
supplements 318–25

Total Daily Energy Expenditure (TDEE) 84, 99, 100, 101, 102, 314, 316, 326

vegan 128, 130, 136, 144, 148, 319
vegetables (fermented), buying & making your own 294–8
vegetarian 121, 132, 148, 319, 345
vitamin supplements 318–19

waist/height ratio 85
weight 60
blueprint for 110–12
influences on 29
plans to achieve ideal 98–105, 313–16
loss 339
loss of & exercise 326

yogurt, buying & making your own 281–3

Recipe Index

5-a-day vegetable and paneer balti 204

Asparagus risotto 248
Avocado toast with feta, lime and chilli 158

Bacon, bean and spinach risotto with white wine 247
Barley pot with balsamic and mustard roast winter roots 232
Beef, mushroom and cashew stir fry 228
Black lentil dal with tomatoes and creamy kefir 214
Blue cheese, leek and potato puff bake 202
Butter bean puttanesca with a baked egg 152

Carrot and coriander soup 186
Cauliflower cheese soup 186
Chicken dirty rice with spices and bacon 206
Chicken pasta bake with ricotta, lemon and veggies 252
Chickpea and leek soup with blue cheese 178
Chilli-spiked vegetarian cottage pie 226
Choc cherry granola 156
Crunchy sweet slaw with dill and caraway 257

Dark chocolate ginger and apricot truffles 268
Dessert black berries parfait pot 266

Egg pancake with quick-blistered veg 191

Fast flatbread pizza 244

Filo tart with brie, winter veg and bacon or mushrooms 222
Filo tart with gruyère, watercress and roast cherry tomato 224
Fuss-free eggs Florentine/Benedict/Royale 164

Greek yogurt fruit sundae with choc-cherry granola 154
Green star minestrone with pesto 176

Heart-warmer porridge with banana, cinnamon and pecans 169
Home-made fresh apple and cabbage sauerkraut 295
Hot artichoke and pepper spread with mozzarella on sourdough
    toast 189
Hot devil 244
Hot lamb meatballs with red slaw and cinna-mint drizzle 234

Kale salad with peas and pesto flavour 259
Kefir 286

Little kefir parfait shot 266

Mexican smoky bean soup with kefir swirl 174
Mexican tomato scramble on toast. Vegan version 171
Middle Eastern spiced bean burgers with halloumi and aubergine
    'buns' 211
Middle Eastern veg 245
Mushroom and black bean koftas with cinna-mint drizzle, red slaw
    and pitta breads 237
Mushroom and tofu/chicken stroganoff 209

Overnight power oats with fruit and crunchy nuts 167

Pink tzatziki with super-fast chickpea flatbread 195
Porcini mushroom and leek risotto 248
Portobello mushroom rarebit with oven-baked tomatoes 150
Pumpkin and lentil soup with herb-infused olive oil 182
Punchy new potato salad with egg and pea shoots 220
Purple sprouting broccoli with Romesco sauce 261

Quick-as-a-flash cauliflower and broccoli tabbouleh 187

Refried beans with white cheese and coriander 255
Revved-up Caesar salad with parmesan and mustard kefir dressing
    200

Smoked salmon spaghetti and courgette with creamy watercress
    sauce 242
Soup (basic recipe) 184
Sourdough 289
Speedy chicken tikka masala 230
Spicy sesame prawn noodle salad 218
Sticky ginger chicken/tofu with turmeric rice noodles 250
Summer berries with kefir cheesecake topping 265
Sweet potato and broad bean tortilla 216
Sweet potato and chilli soup 186
Sweet potato bubble and squeak mash with blue cheese/horseradish
    sauce 162
Sweet potato, lime and turmeric wedges 263

Thyme and sweet pepper hummus with crudités 197
Tomato and strawberry gazpacho 180

vegetables, fermenting 295
Veggie dirty rice with spices and sausages 208

Waldorf muffins with blue cheese, apple and walnuts 160
Warm puy lentil salad with jewel veg and chilli dressing 240
Wedge salad with blue cheese dressing 193

Yogurt 282

Acknowledgements

I couldn't have written *The Dirty Diet* without help from those who gave their time, energy and ideas.

Thanks to the Seven Dials team at Orion – Amanda and Katie for getting behind it; Sarah, Amy and Virginia for helping share the idea with the world. To Helen, Faith and Nikki for making the food look gorgeous. To Alice for attention to detail. And especially to Emily for brilliant editing and juggling so many different deadlines and pressures.

Thanks to Araminta for being a fantastic cheerleader and a huge supporter of the idea and the principles behind it.

Special thanks to Helen Phadnis for being the most down to earth, yet expert, dietitian around – and for being such a huge fan of cheese!

Thanks to Dr Lesley Hoyles for putting me straight on poo, guts and so much more.

Thanks to Frances Reid for sourdough expertise, and to everyone at Loving Foods for talking fermented veggies.

Thanks to my friends for putting up with me banging on about bacteria, especially the Kitties, and to Rich for trying out my recipes and keeping me on track when I thought I'd never get it all done in time.